HEALING THE HEART

DEEPAK CHOPRA, M.D.

*H*EALING THE

*H*EART

a spiritual approach to

reversing coronary artery disease

Harmony Books / New York

Published by Harmony Books, a division of Crown Publishers, Inc., 201 East 50th Street, New York, New York 10022. Member of the Crown Publishing Group.

Random House, Inc. New York, Toronto, London, Sydney, Auckland
www.randomhouse.com

HARMONY and colophon are trademarks of Crown Publishers, Inc.

Printed in the United States of America

Library of Congress Cataloging-in-Publication Data
Chopra, Deepak.
    Healing the heart : a spiritual approach to reversing coronary artery disease / Deepak Chopra.
        p.   cm.
    Includes index.
    1. Coronary heart disease—Alternative treatment.   2. Coronary heart disease—Prevention.   3. Medicine, Ayurvedic.   4. Coronary heart disease—Risk factors.   I. Title.
    RC685.C6C48   1998b
    616.1'23—dc21   97-52794
                                                     CIP

ISBN 0-609-60035-4

10 9 8 7 6 5 4 3 2 1

First Edition

CONTENTS

PART ONE

THE PROBLEM OF CORONARY HEART DISEASE

THE CENTER OF OUR BEING

The human heart exists not only in the middle of our chests, but also in the center of our consciousness. It is the focal point of the human circulatory system, and it is the true seat of the soul. The heart's central role is evident even in our language. Whenever we speak "from the heart," we refer to those issues that are most important to us. We call our deepest feelings for the people we love "matters of the heart." But despite all this, in contemporary society the human heart is often stripped of its poetry. Medical science in particular considers the heart in mostly mechanical terms, like any other piece of machinery—like any other pump.

In our emotional lives we readily associate the heart with our most strongly held feelings, beliefs, and experiences. But if heart disease occurs, we tend to put these aspects of the heart aside; it seems naive to imagine that mere emotions could exert any significant influence on this most central organ of the physical self. But I am convinced that the relationship between mind and body—between head and heart—is just as important to the outcome of heart disease as any medication, diet, or exercise program.

Today we understand that eating steak and eggs every morning or sitting on the couch all day can be dangerous to our health. For a person who wants to avoid a heart attack, changing these habits is important. But lifestyle adjustments are just the beginning. What's essential is a new way of seeing, a quantum leap beyond the conventional model of health, disease, and the human body.

Let me explain exactly what this quantum leap entails. Prior to revolutionary discoveries by Albert Einstein and other physicists early in this century, Western science had been dominated by a mechanistic and materialist view of the universe for more than two hundred years. Since the late seventeenth century, when Isaac Newton formulated the laws of gravity and planetary motion, the cosmos was understood as some vast machine, like a giant clock. The essential task of science was to understand how this machine worked, to describe its operation with accuracy, and to put this knowledge to work benefiting humankind.

The human body, too, was seen by Western science as a complex machine. When disease or injury occurred, Western medicine diagnosed and treated the problem in much the same way that a good mechanic would. Even today this is how most people understand their physical selves.

In the past century a fundamental change in the way physicists think of the universe has had supremely important implications for our understanding of the human body. At the most basic—or quantum—levels, the materialist model of creation has proven inadequate because the material itself has literally disappeared. Subatomic matter is not really matter at all, but fluctuations of energy that merely seem solid if observed under certain conditions. Quantum reality is indistinct, elusive, constantly changing, full of apparent contradictions. What's more, the nature and even the very existence of quantum reality is dependent upon observation. Without an observer, without a consciousness focused on determining what is "there" at the quantum level, nothing is there at all. At the foundation of the universe, therefore, consciousness literally creates reality. The gap between this way of thinking and the old mechanistic view of the universe can only be bridged by a "quantum leap."

In the wake of these developments in modern physics, it has become increasingly clear that the human body is not just a machine made of bone and tissue, but something of a very different order. Our existence as physical beings cannot be understood separately from what we think and feel, because the cells of our flesh and blood are directly and powerfully influenced by our consciousness: *Every thought creates a molecule.* Everything that takes place at the mental, emotional, and spiritual levels of our existence manifests itself at the physical level as well. Who we are physically is not just a matter of how much we weigh or what year we were born. Who we are—and who we choose to become—is also what we think and feel and believe. Health, then, is not just the absence of disease. It is the harmonious integration of our consciousness, our physical selves, and the universe around us. The universe is our extended body, and our bodies contain the universe.

In this book we will explore these new perspectives as they pertain to coronary heart disease. Owing to the serious problem of CHD in our society, this exploration is an extremely important undertaking. Indeed, heart disease is very much on the minds of millions of Americans. Every day new drugs, books, seminars, articles, and research studies announce findings about heart disease. Your cholesterol count is as familiar to you as your phone number. There are heart-healthy cookbooks, heart-wise meal selections in restaurants, and heart monitors to help keep your cardiovascular system under control. Old ideas about heart disease are replaced by new ones, and new ideas are invalidated to give way to timeworn truths.

There are good reasons for our intense interest in the heart.

Heart disease is by far the leading cause of death in the United States. In 1994, heart attacks caused approximately one of every five fatalities in this country. Cardiovascular illness accounts for almost twice as many deaths as result from all types of cancer, and coronary heart disease is specifically responsible for nearly half of all heart-related deaths. Moreover, while cancer is primarily a disease of the elderly, almost half of all heart attacks strike people under the age of sixty-five. About 250,000 of these heart attack victims die within one hour of experiencing symptoms. Perhaps most ominously, approximately 25 percent of all heart attacks strike people who have no known risk factors of any kind.

When heart disease strikes, it brings its victim face-to-face with mortality. If you are recovering from a heart attack, you may suddenly find new restrictions on activities that previously brought you fulfillment and pleasure. Many patients feel they've been robbed of their strength, endurance, and vitality. Statistics demonstrate that heart disease or a heart attack can permanently injure a person's sense of optimism and hopefulness about life, with severe depression occurring in as many as 40 percent of patients.

So there are good reasons for the abundance of material on the heart and heart disease, yet there remains the question of why I am adding to it. Most books on heart disease, after all, are written by cardiologists, while my own specialties are endocrinology and internal medicine.

It is my training in Ayurveda, the traditional healing science of India, that gives me a perspective on medicine which I would like to share with you in this book. Ayurveda teaches that no one knows more about your health than you yourself, provided you've learned to hear and understand the messages your body provides. As an Ayurvedic physician, I believe that I can learn as much, if not more, from finding out about your mind/body type (as we'll see in chapter 3) than I can from your cholesterol count and other diagnostic indicators.

Ayurveda's purpose is the creation of balance among mind, body, and spirit. The lessons of this timeless science are designed to reveal subtle but powerful connections between your physical self, your emotions, and even the routine activities you perform every day. Moreover, this is not simply a philosophical exercise. Understanding these connections, we can then take practical steps to keep you healthy if your physiology is in balance, or to restore you to health as quickly as possible if a disease process has begun.

While Western medicine is unequaled in its ability to provide acute care, Ayurveda seeks to forestall the need for such crisis interventions. By comprehending a patient's innermost nature, an Ayurvedic physician intends not just to suppress symptoms but to create and maintain a state of *perfect health*.

The problem of coronary heart disease is well suited to an Ayurvedic approach. It transcends the limits of medical specialties, and even of medicine itself as it's generally understood in the West. To think meaningfully about heart disease requires dealing not only with topics such as physiology and chemistry but also with beliefs, fears, and faith. A patient's innermost feelings play a central role in living successfully with heart disease, and ultimately in reversing its course.

The importance of this emotional component simply cannot be overestimated. More than thirty years ago, in 1966, a fascinating illustration of this point was published in the *Journal of the American Medical Association*. In the town of Roseto, Pennsylvania, it was noted that the fatality rate due to heart attack was just half that of the rest of the country. While advancing age generally brings higher rates of cardiac fatalities, in Roseto almost no men in the age range of 55 to 64 died of a heart attack. Yet towns nearby had death rates that closely approximated the national average.

Researchers concluded that this remarkable variance from the norm was unrelated to the conventional risk factors, including cigarette smoking or diet. Instead, they found that

the unique values of this community, including a strong work
ethic, great mutual support of neighbors and friends, reverence
and family care of the elderly, and widely shared communal
rituals, played a strong role in resistance to heart disease.

Researchers continued their study of the people of Roseto
into the 1970s and '80s. Over time the society changed, and
traditional values were replaced by more materialistic goals.
Disparities in income grew sharper. Long-standing rituals were
abandoned. Eventually, in Roseto, rates of heart disease climbed
to meet the national average. This sad but significant example illustrates that heart disease involves the spirit as well as
the body.

IMAGES OF THE HEART

As a child, I was intrigued by my heart—by the very idea that
there was something beating rhythmically within my chest,
and that my life would go on as long as this beating continued. Because my father was a physician—a cardiologist, in
fact—I had the opportunity to listen to my heart through a
stethoscope. It was like looking at the stars through a tele-
scope or peering at a blade of grass through a microscope; it
gave me the same awesome sense of being in touch with the
majestic power of the universe.

But there was more. My child's heart seemed attuned to the
ebb and flow of the world around me. I could sense it beating
faster when I was frightened or out of breath, then feel it
returning to normal when I relaxed. Intuitively, I had no doubt
that the heart was the most important organ in the body.
Wasn't it obvious?

Soon enough, however, I learned that the heart was not so
supremely important after all. Elementary school science classes
informed me the brain was the real control center of vital
functions. Although I had believed that the surest indication of

life was the presence of a heartbeat, I now learned that life was present as long as the brain was functioning, and that life ended only when brain activity ceased.

In comparison with the brain's seemingly infinite complexity, the heart was revealed as a simple pumping device, a machine made of muscle. The importance I had instinctively attached to the heart's role turned out to be childish thinking. The intellectual and neurological functions of the brain were the true foundations of human life.

Although I grew up in India, today I can see that this progression of ideas was distinctly Western. The brain is understood to be the repository of factual, scientific knowledge—and our Western society stipulates that information derived from scientific experimentation takes primacy over the mere instincts and emotions that have traditionally been associated with the heart. As the late philosopher of science Paul Feyerabend expressed it, Western culture demands that "we adapt to knowledge in the shape that it is presented by scientists." If our unschooled beliefs don't conform to that outline, it must mean that our beliefs are naive, they're in error, and they'll have to go.

Throughout this book I will suggest that our emphasis on knowledge over belief is a false distinction from the outset. Because of its dual character as the seat of passion and as a mechanical pump, the heart provides an extremely good opportunity for making this point. I believe that our current epidemic of heart disease derives not only from high cholesterol and improper exercise, but from suppressed feeling and ignored intuition.

Since the beginning of civilization, the heart has been the symbol of poetry and spirituality. Those qualities have been devalued by our culture in recent times, and a high incidence of heart disease has been part of the price we've paid. It's hardly surprising, therefore, that the two greatest risk factors for a first heart attack in men under fifty are disliking one's job and a general feeling of unhappiness. I am convinced that by rediscovering our inner wisdom, by reestablishing the powerful connection between mind, body, and emotions, and by making the lifestyle changes suggested in the chapters that follow, coronary heart disease can be prevented and its effects can be reversed when it has already occurred.

YOUR INTEREST IN CHD

I've discussed some of my motivation for writing this book, and I'm sure you have your own reasons for reading about coronary artery disease. It may be that you or someone close to you may have recently had a heart attack, and you're suddenly challenged to learn as much about the heart as you can. Or perhaps you feel you're reaching a point in life when heart trouble is more likely to become a problem and you want to begin taking better care of yourself. Or perhaps you're simply interested in learning more about the mind/body approach to a fundamental area of human health.

You may wish to protect your heart by taking a more active role with your health care providers. You may want to ask more questions, or try new medications, or discontinue some of the medications you're currently taking. Perhaps you want to explore alternative approaches to health care. This desire to take control of your health is important and powerful. As Dr. Bernie Siegel has pointed out in his book *Love, Medicine, and Miracles,* actively engaged patients seem to get better faster.

Regardless of your specific reasons for reading this book, it's unlikely that you are coming to the subject with no prior knowledge. You may already know some of the most important facts about heart disease.

- You may know that, despite the grim statistics cited earlier in this chapter, the number of fatal heart attacks has actually been declining over the past ten years. You may be curious about how this improvement has been achieved, and what it can mean to you.

- Perhaps you've also heard that heart disease may actually be reversible through diet and lifestyle changes, and you're eager to learn more about this possibility.

As a way of beginning the discussion of coronary artery disease that will comprise the rest of this book, I'd like to look in more detail at these two topics.

THE RECENT DECLINE AND WHAT IT MEANS

Heart attacks and cardiovascular disease are the leading causes of death in the United States, but it would be a mistake to limit the scope of the problem to this country. Much has been written about the damaging effects of the typical American diet and lifestyle on cardiovascular health. People in other parts of the world may have been spared these afflictions, possibly because they were closer to nature and therefore purer of heart than residents of the more industrialized nations. But as the way of life followed in the United States and other Western countries spreads across the world—and technological advances are making this happen very quickly—heart disease is becoming a worldwide concern. In India, for example, heart disease is now a leading cause of death.

Coronary heart disease, therefore, is no longer a problem particular to a certain group of people living in a certain place. It is a problem of modern civilization in the largest sense.

As if this spreading epidemic of heart disease were not complicated enough, there is the apparent paradox that the incidence of fatal heart attacks in the United States has been declining over the past ten years. This is certainly encouraging news, but it requires some explanation. This decline is

principally the result of technological innovations on the part
of conventional medicine, as well as the introduction of powerful new medications.

These innovations will be discussed in greater detail in
chapter 6. Right now, however, an important point must be
made. Although many lives have been saved by angiograms,
angioplasty, bypass surgery, and drugs, these are not really solu-
tions to the problem of coronary artery disease. As explained
by the author of the extraordinary book *Dr. Dean Ornish's
Program for Reversing Heart Disease,* invasive procedures
merely interrupt the progression of the disease at the final
stages, with no guarantee that the problems will not recur. In
fact, odds are they almost certainly will.

Our purpose here is to discover ways in which the problem
can be dealt with in its earlier stages, or with less trauma for
the patient. The current statistical improvement is deceptive.
It is true that people are being saved from death, but while
"being saved" is better than dying, it's not really a fundamental solution to the problem. If large numbers of people were
being saved from drowning because of the development of
better life rafts, we would be grateful for lives saved—but it
would be even better if they never fell into the water in the
first place.

THE GOAL: REVERSING CORONARY
HEART DISEASE

It has been convincingly demonstrated that coronary artery
disease may actually be reversible through diet and lifestyle
changes. This is an extremely important fact that has wide
implications for all aspects of health care. When Dr. Dean
Ornish raised this possibility in his book, it became a nation-
wide bestseller, read by millions of people. Yet despite the

success of the book, I don't believe the importance of the breakthrough it represented has been sufficiently understood.

If you were to give a one-sentence summary of the goal of medicine, you might well say something like, "To cure disease." However, the word *cure* is rarely if ever heard in modern medical schools, where the emphasis is on accurately diagnosing and treating illness rather than curing it. Doctors are trained to understand the intricate operations of a disease process, and then to interfere with that process in one way or another. Yet the idea of reversing a disease goes beyond just curing it. Reversal suggests that the disease process is not simply stopped, but that the patient's physiology can be renewed, as if the illness had never done its damage in the first place.

It is also a principle of Vedic philosophy that nothing in Nature is ever final. Nothing is permanent, nothing is created forever, and certainly nothing is ever permanently destroyed. In the chapters that follow, we'll apply this point of view to coronary heart disease, and we'll explore the exciting possibilities that are revealed.

2

PERSPECTIVES ON THE HEART

When I assert that Western medicine is built on a fundamentally materialist concept of the human body, I don't mean to diminish the job that Western doctors perform. Very often, particularly in cases requiring acute care, this approach works extremely well. When someone breaks a bone or needs an appendectomy or requires an MRI scan to locate a tumor, Western medicine provides efficient, effective care.

The materialist orientation, however, is much less successful in preventing disease or in dealing with long-term illness. Here the connection between our health and how we conduct our lives begins to assert itself. When dealing with chronic problems such as coronary heart disease, medicine can no longer separate patients' thoughts and feelings from the paths they must travel toward recovery. Mind/body medicine is built on the premise that any such separation is fundamentally in error.

There may be no other illness in which the connection

between body and mind is so well established as in coronary heart disease. As many as 40 percent of all CHD patients meet the clinical criteria for severe depression. There's nothing mysterious about this; when people are unhappy, they get sick. When they are *heartsick,* literally their hearts are sick.

In the etiology of coronary heart disease, thoughts, feelings, and biology are intimately intertwined. Research shows that clinically depressed people over age fifty-five have a mortality rate four times higher than others, with 63 percent of those deaths coming from heart disease or stroke. Depressed cardiac patients often neglect their medications, perhaps seeing this as a convenient method of suicide.

Every part of our physical being is influenced by—and even created by—our thoughts, feelings, and spiritual aspirations. We now know that emotions spark chemical processes throughout the entire body. Biofeedback research demonstrates that even individual neurons and cells can be influenced by a trained and focused consciousness.

THE HEART AS PUMPING MACHINE

Later in this chapter we will consider the human heart—and by implication the whole body—from a "quantum mechanical" perspective. This view transcends strict divisions between physical matter and energy. It draws upon breakthroughs in quantum physics that have taken place in this century, as well as the traditions of Vedic medicine that have existed for thousands of years.

As a first stop in developing a quantum mechanical perspective, it's important to understand how the heart works as a physical object, and to identify the specific problems that will be the focus of this book.

We know the heart as a single organ, but in some important respects it resembles paired organs of the body, such as the kidneys and the lungs. The right and left sides of the heart, which are joined together by a wall of tissue called the septum, have different tasks and capabilities. The right side of the heart receives oxygen-poor blood that has nourished tissues throughout the body; the right side then pumps this depleted blood the relatively short distance to the lungs, where the blood is infused with new oxygen. The blood then returns to the heart, but to the left side this time, and from here it is pumped back out to nourish the body.

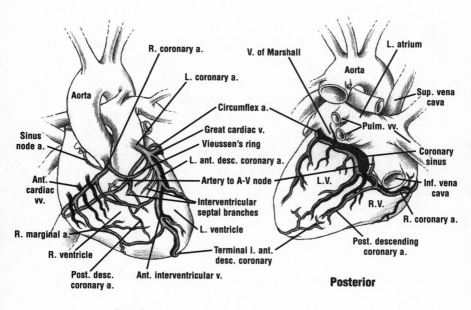

Anterior

Posterior

Both the right and left sides of the heart are divided into upper and lower chambers. The upper areas, called *atria* from the Latin word for chamber, are primarily receiving spaces. The lower areas, called *ventricles,* are the pumping chambers from which the blood is propelled to the rest of the body.

Near the top of the heart, at the right atrium, is a small piece of tissue called the *sinoatrial node*. This tissue functions as a finely tuned power source, a natural pacemaker, which generates an electrical pulse to the heart muscle to control its rhythmic beating. The SA node is the "heart's brain," the center and source of its neural energy. In fact, the heart itself can be compared to a body within a body: like the larger body, this small body is divided into quadrants, with one side stronger than the other. And like the larger body, its brain is located at the top.

There's unmistakable irony in the fact that all the blood that passes through the heart does nothing to nourish the organ itself. Like a bank teller who handles vast sums but earns a relatively small salary, the heart muscle is nourished by a system of arteries that surround the organ in a sort of crown. For this reason, they are called the coronary arteries. The survival of the heart—and the life of its owner—are dependent on these coronary arteries.

Atherosclerosis—that is, blockages of the coronary arteries—is responsible for the majority of heart attacks in the United States. Although many other kinds of problems can affect the heart, the causes, prevention, and reversal of atherosclerosis are the subject of this book.

THE ORIGINS OF CORONARY HEART DISEASE

Coronary heart disease begins with an irritation or injury to the delicate cells that form the lining of the arterial walls. There is much still to be learned about exactly what causes such an injury, but high levels of fat and cholesterol in the bloodstream have been implicated, as have smoking and high blood pressure. Once an injury to the arterial walls has taken place, blood platelets, calcium, and cholesterol begin to build up at the site. Over time a thick plaque forms, narrowing the arterial passageway and reducing the supply of blood to the heart muscle. When pieces of the plaque break off and enter the bloodstream, they can give rise to clots, which can lodge in the narrowed artery and entirely block the flow of blood. This is, quite simply, a heart attack. The vital oxygen supply to a portion of the heart muscle has been cut off, causing the death of the affected area, and often the death of the patient as well.

More than a million Americans will experience a heart attack this year, and half a million will die as a result, roughly ten times the number of American soldiers who died during the entire Vietnam War. In addition, at least 300,000 people in the United States will have coronary bypass operations in an attempt to forestall the complete closure of arteries that have narrowed—operations that typically cost between $50,000 and $100,000 each. Clearly, coronary heart disease exerts a tremendous impact on our society, clinically, emotionally, and financially.

The process of atherosclerosis, described above, can be thought of as a metaphor for the Ayurvedic view of all disease processes. According to Ayurvedic teaching, a healthy human body is like a freely flowing river. Just as a great river is fed by innumerable tributary streams, at every moment our bodies absorb vast amounts of energy and information. Some of this—food, water, or medicine—comes to us in clearly defined physical form, but we also take in sights, sounds, and innumerable other sensations that are difficult to think of in physical terms. Moreover, these incoming packets of information may nourish us, like clear mountain spring water flowing into a major river system, or they may have toxic effects. Just as a river can be slowed or stopped entirely by silt and pollution, disease arises in the human body when toxins overwhelm the system's ability to process them. Flow is replaced by stasis. Healthy circulation is replaced by accumulation. In coronary heart disease, this takes place quite literally. Few medical crises provide such a vivid example of the life force suddenly halted

in its tracks. The process of coronary heart disease is the loss
of natural harmony that characterizes a healthy human body,
a river, a rainforest, a continent, or even the universe as a whole.

Do you feel comfortable with the idea of seeing your body
as a dynamic stream of intelligence, or have you grown attached
to the idea that a human being is largely fixed in time and
space, like a statue? This is not just a philosophical question.
Ayurveda teaches us that consciousness gives rise to reality.
Your view of yourself at this moment directly affects what you
are, right down to the cellular level. By changing your vision
today, you can alter what you will be tomorrow and for the
rest of your life.

Good health begins with awareness of the flowing intelligence that governs your physical body as well as the larger
world in which you live. You can feel this intelligence in your
breathing, in your digestion, in the ebb and flow of energy in
your muscles, and, of course, in the beating of your heart.
Over time, you may have lost touch with this inner awareness,
but regaining it is the first step toward reversing the disease
process. Later in this book you'll learn Ayurvedic techniques
for making this all-important beginning.

THE "RISK FACTOR" APPROACH

Identifying the factors that predispose a person to coronary
heart disease, and then limiting or eliminating those factors, is
clearly a reasonable approach to preventing the illness. As a
medical student, I learned that coronary risk factors included
smoking, high cholesterol, obesity, family history, high blood
pressure, and the extremely competitive, highly stressful personality attributes referred to as Type A behavior. Although
the original formulation of Type A behavior has now been discredited, there are still the major "red flags" for coronary
heart disease, and we will look more closely at each of them

in a subsequent chapter. Another, more recently identified risk factor receiving great attention today is an amino acid found in the blood called homocysteine, derived from animal protein. We will also explore this risk factor in greater depth in chapter 5. But because as many as 25 percent of first heart attacks strike individuals who have no known risk factors, the benefits of this kind of analysis clearly have their limits.

The complexity of dealing with coronary heart disease through risk factor interventions is dramatized by several important studies. In Framingham, Massachusetts, a carefully controlled study of heart disease has been in progress for more than forty years. Some of the data from this study seems clear, especially in regard to blood cholesterol. The chances of a subject developing coronary heart disease, for instance, appears to grow in direct proportion to his or her cholesterol levels. People who had high cholesterol at the beginning of the study proved much more likely to develop coronary heart disease in the future. Conversely, among five thousand men in the study who had cholesterol levels below 150, there was not a single heart attack or death from heart disease for more than twenty-five years. Another major investigation was undertaken by Dr. Larry Scherwitz of the University of California at San Francisco. This study, known as the Multiple Risk Factor Intervention Trial, demonstrated that men aged 35 to 57 with cholesterol counts over 300 were more than four times as likely to die from coronary heart disease as men with levels below 180.

With this information in hand, the next step seems obvious. Subjects should be urged to lower their blood cholesterol by any means necessary, especially the low-density lipoprotein, or LDL, popularly known as "bad cholesterol" owing to its tendency to accumulate in the coronary artery walls. (In contrast, high-density lipoprotein, or HDL, helps cleanse excess cholesterol from the body.) In fact, it seems only logical that people should be told to eliminate other risk factors as well,

such as smoking and consumption of high-fat foods. Yet the
gap between identifying the risk factors and intervention is
greater than one might suppose. In the Framingham study,
subjects who submitted to strictly controlled intervention
showed minimal reduction in heart disease and an overall
increase in mortality.

In researching my book *Ageless Body, Timeless Mind,* I
learned that a similar study had been done in Finland, where
heart attack rates are among the highest in the world. The
study focused on two groups of business executives, all of
whom displayed one or more of the well-documented risk factors for heart disease: obesity, high blood pressure, elevated
cholesterol, and heavy smoking. Over a five-year period, half
of the subjects followed an intensive regimen of controlled
diet, carefully monitoring their condition. The second group,
except for regular checkups, was left entirely unsupervised.

Almost incredibly, death rates from all causes were much
higher among the "healthy living" group during the five years
of the study—with twice as many deaths from heart attacks.
The benefits derived from reduced cholesterol intake and other
lifestyle changes seemed to be more than offset by the stress of
making those adjustments.

Ayurveda teaches that we exist on many levels—physical,
intellectual, emotional, and spiritual. When a person decides
to make changes in his or her life, those changes may be based
on fear, with the drawbacks just discussed. Or change can
have a spiritual source: it may be *inspired* rather than derived
from dread. In my clinical experience this is an extremely significant distinction. Positively based lifestyle changes are much
more likely to yield positive results.

One of my patients in his late thirties, Robert, had been an
outstanding athlete in his youth. Now, however, he had become
quite overweight. He was thinking of taking up jogging and
wanted to consult a physician before starting out.

"Why do you want to become a runner?" I asked.

"To lose weight," Robert replied.

"Yes, but why do you want to lose weight?"

Surprised by my questions Robert disclosed that his boss was threatening to fire him because he'd gotten fat and was projecting a poor corporate image.

I pointed out that this was a questionable reason for embarking on a running program. In fact, given Robert's current physical condition, I believed it might be dangerous to start jogging, given that he would regard it as forced labor. Psychologically and biologically, he might be better off with his current lifestyle.

I was surprised to see a flicker of disappointment in my patient's face when I made this observation. "Perhaps I didn't express myself clearly," I continued. "I'm saying that you don't have to subject yourself to a strenuous exercise program. You can even tell your boss that a doctor advised against it."

The appointment quickly drew to a close. I didn't see Robert again for several years, but one day we met on the street. Physically, the man was completely transformed; he was at least thirty pounds lighter. When I mentioned this, he disclosed that he was now an experienced long-distance runner.

"Well, I can see you didn't take my advice," I remarked. "I imagine your boss must be very pleased."

"Oh, I did take your advice," he said, laughing, "and eventually I got fired. That's when I started running, not to save my job but to get back in touch with the way I used to feel when I was a kid, when I could play sports and exercise for hours without getting tired. Those were some of the happiest moments of my life, and now I can enjoy those feelings again. I actually wanted to start running when I spoke to you in your office, but I'm glad you convinced me not to start for the wrong reasons. I've got a new job, too, and I can honestly say that losing the old one was one of the best things that ever happened to me."

When change comes not from externally generated fears but

from an internal experience of pleasure, positive results are inevitable. It is our nature to seek out joy and avoid pain. Action based on avoidance quickly loses its appeal, but the experience of joy, on the other hand, is self-reinforcing and self-perpetuating. Joy founded in spirit is its own reward.

THE QUANTUM MECHANICAL PERSPECTIVE

The lesson to be learned from the limited success of risk factor interventions is that coronary heart disease is not simply a chemical or biological problem. Rather, it must be approached holistically, with full appreciation of the emotional and even spiritual elements that are involved.

What is the effect of telling people that they must stop smoking or they'll be more likely to have a heart attack? Or that if they don't reduce their blood cholesterol their arteries are inevitably going to become blocked? Or that if they don't lose a significant amount of weight they're much more likely to fall over dead? Quite simply, the risk factors may go down, but the fear levels will significantly elevate—and fear creates stress, which has a significant impact on heart disease.

In order to grasp Ayurveda's approach to coronary heart disease, it's important to understand the Ayurvedic view of who we really are, and of our place in the universe. I often describe this in terms of the quantum mechanical body, a concept that draws on ideas from contemporary physics as well as the insights of traditional Indian medicine.

The quantum mechanical body is comprised of three aspects. Ayurveda refers to these as the physical body, the subtle body, and the causal body. Using the analogy of a computer, these are the printout, the software, and the application of our existence. Matter and energy, localized in space and time, are the components of the physical body. The physical body begins at our conception and disappears at our death when the atoms and molecules of the body disperse. But in fact the physical body is always dispersing, as the atoms of our bodies are constantly being replaced. We literally rebuild ourselves approximately every seven years: Though your form may have remained more or less the same, not one atom in your body today was there less than a decade ago.

Though the physical body reconstructs itself many times during a lifetime before dispersing, the subtle body lasts long after the disappearance of the physical self. The subtle body is composed of thoughts and feelings that exist beyond the limits of the physical world. Beethoven lost his hearing, John Milton lost his sight, but these physical limitations did not prevent the composition of the Ninth Symphony or *Paradise Lost*. And once you've heard the music of Beethoven it will continue to exist in your consciousness regardless of whatever changes your physical body might undergo.

I remember being moved by something I read in a biography of Albrecht Dürer, the great German artist of the fifteenth century. The inscription on his tomb reads, "Whatever was mortal about Dürer is buried here." By implication, his subtle body—the thoughts and ideas and emotions he conveyed through his work and his life—are still very much alive in the world.

Beyond the subtle body is the causal body, a unity of perfect order that encompasses all space-time events. In a way it is analogous to the genetic programming from which the nature of each individual is derived. By interacting with itself in an infinite variety of forms, the causal body is responsible for all of creation. It is the great sea of energy and intelligence from which everything begins and to which everything eventually returns. It is spaceless, timeless, dimensionless. It is both subject and object. At every instant, it is the knower, the process of knowing, and what is known. It is difficult to express the nature of the causal body in everyday language, but two forms of expression come close to conveying its true nature. One is

great poetry, especially classical Vedic texts such as the Upa-
nishads. The other is the elegant mathematical equations of
modern physics, which also seek to convey a reality that transcends the limits of our everyday thoughts and senses.

Ayurveda sees all of creation as a vast interconnecting network of energy and information—flowing, constantly changing,
with each element affecting all the others and even the most
minute events influencing the whole. The heart is not just a
pump whose well-being depends on the fuel that's put into it.
Every aspect of your experience has an effect on your heart,
from the temperature of the room you're in to the kinds of
thoughts that pass through your mind. The condition of your
heart helps define who you are, and who you are determines
the condition of your heart. It should be clear, then, that genuine self-awareness is essential to maintaining a healthy heart,
to recognizing heart disease in its early stages, and to reversing the disease process.

It is inspiring—perhaps even exciting—to approach heart
disease from such an all-encompassing perspective. In discov-
ering new options for healing your heart, I hope that you will
also discover a new way of understanding who you are now
and who you have the power to become.

In the next chapter, we'll learn some of the Ayurvedic principles for achieving this quality of profound self-awareness.

3

KNOWING WHO YOU ARE

I've often noticed that many young children seem to have almost photographic memories, especially for names and faces. A four-year-old, for instance, can recall the identity of someone he or she has met only once, perhaps a year or more in the past, even if her parents have no recollection of the meeting.

To some extent this may be because a child simply doesn't have as much to remember as an adult. But it may also be that children simply see more clearly whatever comes into view. What children see enters a consciousness relatively uncluttered by past association or expectation, so things are seen for what they are. Each person's name, voice, and face is registered as wholly unique.

Every person's face really *is* unique. With the exception of identical twins, no one looks exactly like anyone else. Although it seems almost incredible, as the number of variations would seem to be limited by the number of human facial features, no one who's ever lived looks exactly like any other human being, back to the dawn of history.

People's faces, then, are like snowflakes. No two are the same. According to Ayurvedic teaching, this uniqueness extends to every aspect of our being, including our hearts. Understanding what is unique about ourselves, as well as which characteristics we share with others, is the first critical step toward creating physical, emotional, and spiritual health.

From a healer's point of view, the ability to recognize individual differences and group similarities is also vitally important. When a musician begins playing a Beethoven sonata, she instinctively calls upon and integrates her knowledge of Beethoven's music with every other piece she's ever played. Together with this, she brings an awareness of the specific instrument she's now playing, the size of the concert hall, and the other selections on the program. She recognizes that every performance is unique, but she also understands the need for context. This is really what it means to be a creative artist, whether the creation is beautiful music or perfect health. The science of healing can make use of MRI scans and DNA analysis, but the art must rely on the inner gifts of the physician and of the patient.

PERCEPTIONS AND DISTORTIONS

Suppose you've been feeling very tired for the past few weeks and you don't know why. You're out of breath after even minor exertions, such as lifting a box or climbing a short flight of stairs. You decide to make an appointment with a doctor. Since you haven't seen a physician for a number of years, you ask friends and family members for recommendations, and eventually you schedule a date and time for an examination.

Undoubtedly, your appointment time falls in between other

obligations in a busy schedule. You're eager to see the doctor when you arrive for your appointment, but first you're asked to fill out a medical history form. Then you sit in a waiting room, leafing through magazines. Then a nurse shows you into an examining room, tells you that the doctor will be with you in a few moments, and leaves. The door closes. You sit down on the edge of the examining table. The table is quite tall, so your feet don't reach the floor, just as a child's feet dangle from a chair at the dinner table. Then you wait again.

Does this sound familiar? If you're like most people, you can probably recite from memory the bleak list of objects present in a typical examining room: the scale, the box of tissues, the slot for waste materials with its stenciled warning of BIOHAZARD, and the magazines in a rack on the back of the closed door.

In this scenario, a unique human being becomes a generic patient. More specifically, the sense of anxiety, frustration, displacement, and regression that begins the moment one enters a doctor's office may make clear communication more difficult. The patient may forget to talk about important symptoms or may have a hard time retaining information discussed at the time of the visit. Tension may even have an impact on the patient's vital signs, such as heart rate, blood pressure, and respiration.

Most physicians, pressed by time and the need to cover their overhead, are happy to transform the patient as soon as possible into columns of numbers on a chart. In a typical first meeting, a physician listens for a few moments to a patient's problem, and then says, "Well, I'd like to run some tests." In other words, the doctor believes he will derive greater insights from figures on a page than from the patient sitting on the examining table. And frequently he might be right, because so many patients have lost the ability to hear and understand what their own bodies are telling them.

DEFINITIONS OF DIAGNOSIS

The purpose of diagnostic tests is to identify any illness as precisely as possible. Western medicine places great emphasis on this accurate and detailed diagnosis. Once an illness has presented itself in the form of manifest symptoms, Western medicine draws upon its immense resources to categorize the disease and, it is hoped, interfere with the disease process.

In the Ayurvedic tradition, the word *diagnosis* has a very different meaning. Diagnosis, to an Ayurvedic physician, means knowing and understanding the patient, not the disease. When the true nature of the patient is known—and only then—an illness can also be understood and treated at the most fundamental level.

Even more important, a genuine understanding of a patient's mind/body system can prevent imbalances from ever reaching the point where symptoms become manifest. This, to me, is the highest form of health care: not just treating a patient's illness, but helping the person to live in such a way that illness never occurs in the first place.

The Ayurvedic approach to creating health, therefore, begins with a simple question: Who are you? This doesn't mean only "What hurts?" or "What is your disease?" It means: What is your unique physical, emotional, and spiritual makeup? How has the energy and information of the universe come together in your flesh and blood, in your hopes and dreams? How does this affect your work, your relationships, the kind of foods you eat, the ways you react to stress, even the times you go to sleep at night and wake up in the morning? What makes you different from other people, and what do you share with them? What are your innate strengths and weaknesses? According to Ayurveda, the answers to all these questions can be expressed in terms of your individual constitution, your unique mind/body type.

THE THREE DOSHAS: VATA, PITTA, KAPHA

Ayurveda expresses the similarities and differences among people in terms of three metabolic body types known as *doshas.* Each of us is born with a unique proportion of these doshas, which creates who we are physically, intellectually, and emotionally. Your body type reveals your biochemical individuality, your own unique nature. Corresponding to the body types are prescriptions for diet, exercise, and lifestyle that best suit each individual and maintain balance in your mind/body system.

Although the proportion of the doshas in our makeup can fluctuate to some extent depending on what's going on in our lives, most people have one or two doshas that are most active, while the third remains less so. According to Ayurvedic teaching, a person is "in balance" when the doshas are present in their original proportions, or close to it. But if stress or other causes lead to pronounced deviation from the balance point set at birth, we become increasingly vulnerable to both physical illness and emotional instability. Other factors that may lead to imbalances include our regular habits like how we eat or drink and the way we choose to relax, changes in the season, internal or external trauma, or genetics.

The three doshas are known as *Vata, Pitta,* and *Kapha.*

• **Vata dosha** is the principle of movement that propels our physical systems, such as breathing and circulation. Ayurveda associates Vata with the wind, unpredictable and always in motion. If Vata is dominant in your constitution, you are most likely of slender build, with quick physical gestures and with an equally rapid progression of thoughts and feelings continually passing through your mind. Intensity and constant change are the hallmarks of your daily experience. When a Vata-dominant person's mind/body system is in balance, he or

she is vibrant, creative, and enthusiastic. But if Vata begins to
exceed its normal proportion, there may be anxiety, sleep and
skin disorders, and poor digestion.

• **Pitta dosha** is associated with fire. This dosha controls all
aspects of metabolism, from the digestion of food to the ability to thoroughly process ideas. Pitta dosha is associated with
fire. Pitta-dominant people tend to be of medium build, with
well-proportioned limbs and rather muscular bodies. Often
they have light brown or red hair, with fair skin and blue
eyes. When their systems are in balance, Pittas are warm, intel-
ligent, and insightful. They are often leaders in their careers.
Out-of-balance Pittas can be critical of others, overly competitive, and excessively resentful of perceived slights. "Hot"
emotions, such as anger or impatience, generally derive from
excessive Pitta.

• **Kapha dosha** governs the body's structure and fluid balance. At the microscopic level, Kapha holds the cells together;
expressed on a larger scale, Kapha governs the creation and
maintenance of muscles, bone, and cartilage. Ayurveda associates Kapha with earth, which is the raw material from which
things grow, and with water, which makes earth fertile and
malleable. Kapha-dominant people are often large-boned and
heavyset. Their hair is usually thick and dark. Both in their
thoughts and movements, they are deliberate, calm, and predictable. When balanced, the Kapha nature is characterized by
sweetness, loyalty, and slowness to anger. When excessive,
Kaphas can be inflexible and overbearing. Physically, unbalanced Kaphas are prone to lethargy and overweight.

IDENTIFYING YOUR MIND/BODY TYPE

The questionnaire below is designed to provide a preliminary
indication of your doshic constitution. This can be an important first step toward true awareness of who you really are and

what your needs might be. Identifying your dominant dosha, however, is neither an exact science nor a fortune-telling technique. It's not like casting a horoscope, and it's not like gene mapping, either. Instead, learning your doshic makeup allows you to locate yourself within Ayurveda, an insightful and practical medical system that has benefited humanity for thousands of years. This tradition provides a clear and even poetic vocabulary for describing yourself and your physical, emotional, and spiritual requirements. But it would be a mistake to think that this questionnaire provides an extremely precise description of yourself, or that any application of the doshic terminology should be pushed too far. Vata, Pitta, and Kapha are more than metaphors—Ayurveda teaches that they do exist on the physical level—but they can't be "read" with exactitude, the way, for instance, the temperature of the body can be read from a thermometer.

The determination of your body type is just the beginning of an Ayurvedic approach to restoring health. In Ayurveda, diagnoses of imbalances in your system (that is, disease) are commonly made through examination of the pulse, tongue, eyes, and nails. Treatments may involve a combination of diet, exercise, meditation, breathing exercises, and herbal treatments.

For a more complete and accurate evaluation of your doshic makeup, I recommend consultation with an Ayurvedically trained physician, or a visit to the Chopra Center for Well Being in La Jolla, California.

AYURVEDA MIND/BODY QUESTIONNAIRE

The following quiz is divided into three sections. For the first 20 questions, which apply to Vata dosha, read each statement and choose a response from 0 to 6.

    0 = Doesn't apply to me
    3 = Applies to me somewhat (or some of the time)
    6 = Applies to me mostly (or nearly all of the time)

At the end of the section, write down your total Vata score. For example, if you mark a 6 for the first question, a 3 for the second, and a 2 for the third, your total up to that point would be 6 + 3 + 2 = 11. Total the entire section in this way, and you will arrive at your final Vata score. Proceed to the 20 questions for Pitta and those for Kapha.

When you are finished, you will have three separate scores. Comparing these will determine your body type.

For fairly objective physical traits, your choice will usually be obvious. For mental traits and behavior, which are more subjective, you should answer according to how you have felt and acted most of your life, or at least for the past few years.

SECTION 1: VATA							
	Does not apply		Applies sometimes			Applies most times	
1. I perform activities very quickly.	0	1	2	3	4	5	6
2. I am not good at memorizing things and then remembering them later.	0	1	2	3	4	5	6
3. I am enthusiastic and vivacious by nature.	0	1	2	3	4	5	6
4. I have a thin physique—I don't gain weight very easily.	0	1	2	3	4	5	6
5. I have always learned new things very quickly.	0	1	2	3	4	5	6
6. My characteristic gait while walking is light and quick.	0	1	2	3	4	5	6
7. I tend to have difficulty making decisions.	0	1	2	3	4	5	6
8. I tend to develop gas and become constipated easily.	0	1	2	3	4	5	6
9. I tend to have cold hands and feet.	0	1	2	3	4	5	6
10. I become anxious or worried frequently.	0	1	2	3	4	5	6
11. I don't tolerate cold weather as well as most people do.	0	1	2	3	4	5	6

	Does not apply		Applies sometimes			Applies most times	
12. I speak quickly and my friends think that I'm talkative.	0	1	2	3	4	5	6
13. My moods change easily and I am somewhat emotional by nature.	0	1	2	3	4	5	6
14. I often have difficulty falling asleep or having a sound night's sleep.	0	1	2	3	4	5	6
15. My skin tends to be very dry, especially in winter.	0	1	2	3	4	5	6
16. My mind is very active, sometimes restless, but also very imaginative.	0	1	2	3	4	5	6
17. My movements are quick and active; my energy tends to come in bursts.	0	1	2	3	4	5	6
18. I am easily excitable.	0	1	2	3	4	5	6
19. I tend to be irregular in my eating and sleeping habits.	0	1	2	3	4	5	6
20. I learn quickly, but I also forget quickly.	0	1	2	3	4	5	6

VATA SCORE

SECTION 2: PITTA

	Does not apply		Applies sometimes			Applies most times	
1. I consider myself to be very efficient.	0	1	2	3	4	5	6
2. In my activities, I tend to be extremely precise and orderly.	0	1	2	3	4	5	6
3. I am strong-minded and have a somewhat forceful manner.	0	1	2	3	4	5	6
4. I feel uncomfortable or become easily fatigued in hot weather— more so than other people.	0	1	2	3	4	5	6

	Does not apply		Applies sometimes			Applies most times	
5. I tend to perspire easily.	0	1	2	3	4	5	6
6. Even though I might not always show it, I become irritable or angry quite easily.	0	1	2	3	4	5	6
7. If I skip a meal or a meal is delayed, I become uncomfortable.	0	1	2	3	4	5	6
8. One or more of the following characteristics describes my hair: • early graying or balding • thin, fine, straight • blond, red, or sandy-colored	0	1	2	3	4	5	6
9. I have a strong appetite; if I want to, I can eat quite a large quantity.	0	1	2	3	4	5	6
10. Many people consider me stubborn.	0	1	2	3	4	5	6
11. I am very regular in my bowel habits—it would be more common for me to have loose stools than to be constipated.	0	1	2	3	4	5	6
12. I become impatient very easily.	0	1	2	3	4	5	6
13. I tend to be a perfectionist about details.	0	1	2	3	4	5	6
14. I get angry quite easily, but then I quickly forget about it.	0	1	2	3	4	5	6
15. I am very fond of cold foods, such as ice cream, and also ice-cold drinks.	0	1	2	3	4	5	6
16. I am more likely to feel that a room is too hot than too cold.	0	1	2	3	4	5	6
17. I don't tolerate foods that are very hot and spicy.	0	1	2	3	4	5	6
18. I am not as tolerant of disagreement as I should be.	0	1	2	3	4	5	6

	Does not apply		Applies sometimes		Applies most times	
19. I enjoy challenges, and when I want something I am very determined in my efforts to get it.	0	1	2	3	4	5	6
20. I tend to be quite critical of others and also of myself.	0	1	2	3	4	5	6

PITTA SCORE

SECTION 3: KAPHA

	Does not apply		Applies sometimes		Applies most times	
1. My natural tendency is to do things in a slow and relaxed fashion.	0	1	2	3	4	5	6
2. I gain weight more easily than most people and lose it more slowly.	0	1	2	3	4	5	6
3. I have a placid and calm disposition—I'm not easily ruffled.	0	1	2	3	4	5	6
4. I can skip meals easily without any significant discomfort.	0	1	2	3	4	5	6
5. I have a tendency toward excess mucus or phlegm, chronic congestion, asthma, or sinus problems.	0	1	2	3	4	5	6
6. I must get at least eight hours of sleep in order to be comfortable the next day.	0	1	2	3	4	5	6
7. I sleep very deeply.	0	1	2	3	4	5	6
8. I am calm by nature and not easily angered.	0	1	2	3	4	5	6
9. I don't learn as quickly as some people, but I have excellent retention and a long memory.	0	1	2	3	4	5	6

	Does not apply		Applies sometimes			Applies most times	
10. I have a tendency toward becoming plump—I store extra fat easily.	0	1	2	3	4	5	6
11. Weather that is cool and damp bothers me.	0	1	2	3	4	5	6
12. My hair is thick, dark, and wavy.	0	1	2	3	4	5	6
13. I have smooth, soft skin with a somewhat pale complexion.	0	1	2	3	4	5	6
14. I have a large, solid body build.	0	1	2	3	4	5	6
15. The following words describe me well: serene, sweet-natured, affectionate, and forgiving.	0	1	2	3	4	5	6
16. I have slow digestion, which makes me feel heavy after eating.	0	1	2	3	4	5	6
17. I have very good stamina and physical endurance as well as a steady level of energy.	0	1	2	3	4	5	6
18. I generally walk with a slow, measured gait.	0	1	2	3	4	5	6
19. I have a tendency toward oversleeping and grogginess upon awakening, and am generally slow to get going in the morning.	0	1	2	3	4	5	6
20. I am a slow eater and am slow and methodical in my actions.	0	1	2	3	4	5	6

KAPHA SCORE

FINAL SCORE

VATA   **PITTA**   **KAPHA**

HOW TO DETERMINE YOUR BODY TYPE

Now that you have added up your scores, you can determine your body type. Although there are only three doshas, remember that Ayurveda combines them in ten ways to arrive at ten different body types.

- **If one score is much higher than the others, you are probably a single-dosha type.**

  Single-Dosha Types
  Vata
  Pitta
  Kapha

You are definitely a single-dosha type if your highest score is twice as high as the next highest dosha score (for instance, Vata—90, Pitta—45, Kapha—35). In single-dosha types, the characteristics of Vata, Pitta, or Kapha predominate. Your next highest dosha may still show up in your natural tendencies, but it will be much less distinct.

- **If no single dosha dominates, you are a two-dosha type.**

  Two-Dosha Types
  Vata-Pitta or Pitta-Vata
  Pitta-Kapha or Kapha-Pitta
  Vata-Kapha or Kapha-Vata

If you are a two-dosha type, the traits of your two leading doshas will predominate. The higher one comes first in your body type, but both count.

Most people are two-dosha types. A two-dosha type might have a score like this: Vata—80, Pitta—90, Kapha—20. If this was your score, you would consider yourself to be a Pitta-Vata type.

- **If your three scores are nearly equal, you may be a three-dosha type.**

  Three-Dosha Type
  Vata-Pitta-Kapha

However, this type is considered rarest of all. Check your answers again, or have a friend go over your responses with you. Also, you can read over the descriptions of Vata, Pitta, and Kapha on pages 31–32 to see if one or two doshas are more prominent in your makeup.

INTERPRETING YOUR RESULTS

By identifying and understanding your body type, you can gain insight into your genuine needs, as distinct from the often self-destructive impulses that arise from stress, fear, or other negative sources. You may experience a profound sense of recognition, or even a feeling of acceptance for traits that you may not have previously appreciated. Learning about the doshas may also give you insight into differences between yourself and others who are close to you. The lists below provide a shorthand summary of the dosha characteristics. With your questionnaire results in mind, do you recognize many of these traits in yourself? Are they in accord with your dominant dosha, as indicated by the questionnaire?

Vata Characteristics

- Light, thin build
- Performs activity quickly
- Irregular hunger and digestion
- Light, interrupted sleep; tendency toward insomnia
- Enthusiasm, vivacity, imagination
- Excitability, changing moods
- Quick to grab new information, also quick to forget
- Tendency to worry
- Tendency to be constipated
- Tires easily, tendency to overexert
- Mental and physical energy comes in bursts

Vata-dominant people often . . .

- Feel hungry at any time of the day or night
- Love excitement and constant change
- Go to sleep at different times every night, skip meals, and keep irregular habits in general
- Digest food well one day and poorly the next
- Display bursts of emotion that are short-lived and quickly forgotten
- Walk quickly

Pitta Characteristics

- Medium build
- Medium strength and endurance
- Sharp hunger and thirst, strong digestion
- Tendency to become angry or irritable under stress
- Fair or ruddy skin, often freckled
- Aversion to sun, hot weather
- Enterprising character, likes challenges
- Sharp intellect
- Precise, articulate speech
- Cannot skip meals
- Blond, light brown, or red hair (or reddish undertones)

Pitta-dominant people often . . .

- Feel ravenous if dinner is half an hour late
- Live by their watches and resent having their time wasted
- Wake up at night feeling hot and thirsty
- Take command of a situation or feel that they should
- Find others feel they are too demanding, sarcastic, or critical
- Walk with a determined stride

Kapha Characteristics

- Solid, powerful build; great physical strength and endurance
- Steady energy; slow and graceful in action
- Tranquil, relaxed personality; slow to anger
- Cool, smooth, thick, pale, and often oily skin
- Slow to grasp new information, but good retentive memory
- Heavy, prolonged sleep
- Tendency toward obesity
- Slow digestion, mild hunger
- Affectionate, tolerant, forgiving
- Tendency to be possessive, complacent

Kapha-dominant people often . . .

- Mull things over for a long time before making a decision
- Wake up slowly, lie in bed a long time, and need coffee upon rising
- Are satisfied with the status quo and preserve it by conciliating others
- Respect other people's feelings (with which they feel genuine empathy)
- Seek emotional comfort in food
- Move gracefully, with a gliding walk, even if overweight

Understanding the profound influence of the doshas both physically and emotionally is the foundation of the Ayurvedic approach to living in balance. With this understanding, you can answer that first, all-important question—"Who are you?"—in a way that reveals both the uniqueness of your own being and your oneness with all of creation. With this understanding, you can nurture and strengthen yourself, and share this strength with everyone who is in your life.

In the next chapter we will explore the ways that imbalances in the doshas, particularly as they relate to the emotions, can affect the health of your heart. As we've discussed, psychology and biology are intricately intertwined. By unraveling the knots in your emotional body, you can begin to remove barriers to wellness and alter the course of disease.

4

CORONARY HEART DISEASE

AND THE EMOTIONS

When I was in medical school, there was a growing recognition of the role that personality plays in the development of heart disease. Although no hard data existed to support the idea, heart attacks just seemed more likely to happen to tense, high-strung individuals than to those who were more placid.

This led to the concept of the Type-A personality: a hard-driving, competitive, deadline-oriented, frequently angry, highly demanding individual. Since it seemed that Type-A personalities were at high risk for heart attacks, programs were instituted to reduce Type-A behavior. Unfortunately, the number of heart attacks went up rather than down—and today no one believes that Type-A behavior as it was originally described is a cause of heart attacks. Research does seem to indicate, however, that the way you react to stress can be a factor in the development of heart disease.

Despite the fact that the attempt to link heart disease to personality has been inconclusive, I believe the idea is fundamentally sound and extremely important. New research supports this belief. A four-year study of middle-aged men who expressed hopelessness about the future found a 20 percent greater increase in the narrowing of coronary arteries than was found in more optimistic individuals. This is approximately the same magnitude of increase as results from smoking a pack of cigarettes every day. Although it is not clear exactly how hopelessness hastens coronary artery disease, the researchers noted that psychological factors can affect the production of stress hormones, which may work to constrict the arterial passageways. In times of stress, your heart rate and blood pressure rise, increasing your heart's need for oxygen. Hormones released in times of stress can damage the arterial walls and also increase cholesterol levels and raise blood pressure. In people with heart disease, stress reactions and emotional upsets can lead to angina or even a heart attack.

Other emotional issues can affect the health of your heart. Research has shown that people who are isolated, or those who have experienced multiple stressful life events, such as a death in the family, a divorce, or even a job change, may be at higher risk for heart disease.

THE AYURVEDIC VIEW OF STRESS

From an Ayurvedic viewpoint, stress is an experience of imbalance. Whether it is brought on by a physical event or an emotion, stress occurs when a person is unable to receive information into the mind/body system in a balanced way.

Many of life's stresses, though hardly dramatic when viewed as separate incidents, nevertheless take their toll on us as they are repeated over and over again. Many people are all too familiar with the corrosive quality of emotional stress caused by irritating work problems experienced on a regular basis. And while most of our greatest joys may come from our connection to family, some of the most stressful moments in our lives may arise when we find ourselves at odds with those who matter most to us. While our bodies have finely tuned systems capable of handling high levels of stress from time to time, we are not made to endure it on a prolonged basis. To do so harms the heart in both its emotional and its physical aspects.

At every moment, every cell in your body is hard at work nourishing itself, defending itself, and repairing damage. But under great stress, the cells actually stop this process of renewal as they are called upon to perform a range of other activities to meet situational demands. Every cell in your body is filled with infinite intelligence, including the intelligence to heal and reverse disease. So it is important that we do all we can to ensure that our own stress reactions aren't so severe that they hinder one of our most basic mechanisms for health and healing.

Over many centuries, the relationship between personality and illness has been studied and refined in Ayurveda. This connection is particularly important in coronary heart disease, where emotions associated with each of the three doshas have specific effects on the progress of the illness. The information that follows can help you to identify imbalances in your system related to the emotions. You are unique in your reactions to life, and a lot can be learned about who you are and what you need to regain your balance, simply by evaluating how you feel and behave in certain situations.

HEART DISEASE AND UNBALANCED VATA

Vata dosha is characterized by sudden change and unpredictability. Although Vata imbalance is associated with several forms of heart problems, including palpitations and arrhythmias, it is generally less significant in coronary heart disease than Pitta or Kapha imbalance.

Symptoms of Vata-related heart disease include shortness of

breath, dry cough, and fainting. Insomnia, unhealthy diet, and
an inability to relax are common Vata behaviors that can
exacerbate the problem. Although your results on the Mind/
Body Questionnaire may not have identified Vata as your
dominant dosha, your current condition may still be characterized by a Vata imbalance. Answering the ten questions below
will help you determine the extent to which such an imbalance
is present in your physiology.

For each question, respond with a number from 1 through 5
that best reflects your feelings, as described in the scale below:

    1 = Not at all
    2 = Slightly
    3 = Somewhat
    4 = Moderately
    5 = Extremely

 1. I like to gossip.
 2. I have trouble making up my mind when ordering in a
    restaurant.
 3. I like to engage strangers in conversation.
 4. I tend to bolt when I feel hurt.
 5. I often misplace my keys, wallet, or pocketbook.
 6. People remind me of things I've said that I don't
    remember.
 7. In relationships, I tend to be "high maintenance."
 8. I eat and sleep on irregular schedules.
 9. My feelings are easily hurt.
10. My moods change easily and quickly.

If your responses total 50 or close to it, your current condition is characterized by unbalanced Vata dosha. A vital key to
reestablishing balance is the development of a stable, struc-
tured lifestyle, with regular routines and predictable schedules.
If you're a Vata-dominant type, this may go against your nat-

ural instincts. You may feel more at home with a lifestyle that others would consider little short of chaotic. But it is important to break out of this apparent comfort zone if balance is to be restored. By stabilizing what you do during the day, you'll also stabilize how you feel. And your heart, in turn, will become less subject to erratic and dangerous episodes.

The daily routine described later in this chapter is especially important and beneficial for pacifying out-of-balance Vata.

HEART DISEASE AND UNBALANCED PITTA

Although the connection between so-called Type-A personality and heart disease has been largely discredited, one behavioral component of Type-A continues to be viewed as a significant factor. This is a pattern of generalized hostility and continuing, free-floating anger.

From an Ayurvedic point of view, this is significant information. Anger is a hot emotion. Your face turns red when you're angry, and you may suddenly begin to perspire as though you were running a high fever. Since Pitta dosha is associated with fire and heat, Ayurveda describes chronic anger and hostility as arising primarily from a Pitta imbalance. Moreover, since coronary heart disease arises out of an irritation or inflammation of the arterial walls, CHD can be understood as a Pitta-related illness.

Pitta-dominant people typically feel an especially strong need to be in control. They are orderly and precise, with strong powers of concentration and sharp intellects. They persevere in a task until they feel mastery has been achieved. They are very punctual. They take responsibility seriously, both in their work and their personal lives. They don't like to miss a deadline, whether it's for a business presentation or serving a meal. By instinct, Pittas are clean, well-organized, and highly efficient.

In general, these are positive characteristics—but they can become destructive when Pitta accumulates to excess. Perfectionism, compulsive behavior, impatience, and hostile judgments of others are characteristic of unbalanced Pitta. There is a need to assert total mastery over oneself, over other people, and over the world in general. Since that level of complete control is impossible to achieve, a sense of frustration builds up, which expresses itself in the generalized hostility characteristic of Pitta imbalance. This can significantly raise the risk of coronary heart disease.

The questions below will help identify the presence of out-of-balance Pitta. Use the scale below to assess your level of agreement with each statement:

1 = Not at all
2 = Slightly
3 = Somewhat
4 = Moderately
5 = Extremely

1. Under pressure, the easiest emotion for me to show is anger.
2. I carry resentment for the way I've been treated by people in the past.
3. In my house, people are expected to follow the rules.
4. I'm sometimes seen as sarcastic or cynical.
5. I do not tolerate sloppy work.
6. I expect people to be on time for appointments.
7. I have a low threshold for tolerating noise.
8. In relationships, I believe that one person gets more than the other.
9. I feel upset when my meals don't occur on a regular schedule.
10. I blame my parents for many of my current problems.

A total of 50 or close to it suggests that being in control is a highly important need for you. It's also likely that you're angry that this need is not being fully satisfied. As a first step toward dealing with the Pitta imbalance that underlies these feelings, read the seven-step program that appears at the end of this chapter. These are actions you can take right now to benefit your overall physical and emotional well-being, and the health of your heart in particular.

HEART DISEASE AND UNBALANCED KAPHA

Kapha-dominant people are naturally slow and easygoing. Unlike Pittas, they are not particularly attached to tight schedules and planned routines in their everyday lives. They tend to be tolerant and forgiving, and they will put up with unpleasantness for long periods before becoming angry. The general slowness of their natures, however, means that Kaphas are retentive individuals. They require long periods of time to process an experience, whether it's a heavy meal or a perceived insult. High blood cholesterol is a common Kapha-related problem, both because Kaphas tend to eat rich foods and because their systems are slow to metabolize the residues of such a diet. This same sluggishness can express itself in the emotional lives of Kapha types as well. They may hold on to hurts, betrayals, and disappointments; this can create toxic feelings of hostility just as undigested foods can give rise to toxins in the body.

To determine the extent to which unbalanced Kapha may be responsible for emotional difficulties in your life, answer the questions below with a number 1 through 5, using the scale established earlier.

1. I am happier working alone than with others.
2. I like to remind people of all that I've done for them.

  3. I tend to harbor old hurts.
  4. I withdraw if I feel slighted.
  5. I'm good at caring for other people's needs.
  6. If something's bothering me, I keep it to myself.
  7. I don't need to be liked by everyone.
  8. I often oversleep.
  9. Confrontations make me uncomfortable.
 10. I feel hurt if friends and family don't regularly call me.

A Kapha imbalance is indicated if your responses total close to 50. Although Kapha-dominant people are naturally easygoing and even-tempered, unbalanced Kaphas are subject to a wide range of destructive emotions, including depression, procrastination, and self-pity. To restore balance, it's important to overcome inertia and get moving, both physically and emotionally. The daily routine below can serve as a starting point for overcoming sedentary tendencies. Particular attention should be given to exercise, massage, and the importance of going to bed and awakening at early hours.

YOUR DAILY ROUTINE

According to Ayurvedic teaching, each day unfolds according to a natural rhythm. By synchronizing your daily routine with these natural ebbs and flows, and by living each moment mindfully and completely, you can bring health to your body and joy to your spirit. This is true regardless of your mind/body type, but it's especially important when your system has become unbalanced.

This schedule can help you align your daily activities with Nature's rhythms.

Morning: 6:00 to 8:00 A.M.

- Wake without an alarm clock.
- Brush your teeth and clean your tongue if coated.
- Drink a glass of warm water to encourage regular elimination.
- Empty your bowels and bladder.
- Massage your body, either with oil or dry massage. For detailed discussion of massage and the heart, see chapter 9.
- Bathe.
- Perform light exercise. For further discussion, see chapter 8.
- Meditate. For further discussion, see chapter 7.
- Eat breakfast.
- Take a midmorning walk.

Afternoon: Noon to 1:00 P.M.

- Eat lunch (the largest meal of the day).
- Sit quietly for five minutes after eating.
- If possible, take a short walk to aid digestion.
- Meditate in the late afternoon.

Evening: 6:00 to 7:00 P.M.

- Eat a light to moderate dinner.
- Sit quietly for five minutes after eating.
- Walk for five to fifteen minutes to aid digestion.

Bedtime: 9:30 to 10:30 P.M.

- Perform light activity in the evening.
- Go to bed early, but at least three hours after dinner.
- Do not read, eat, or watch TV in bed.

METABOLIZING AND RELEASING
EMOTIONAL TOXINS

Ayurveda teaches us to live in the present moment, unencumbered by regrets from the past or worries about the future. Just as the healthy body completely digests a meal, the healthy spirit has the power to thoroughly process experiences, allowing us to freely move ahead with our lives. But for most people, this is more easily said than done. Our hearts, both literally and figuratively, are congested with anger, doubt, and fear.

If your system has lost the ability to thoroughly process your experiences, you can take specific steps to restore that power. Later in this book we'll discuss those steps in terms of diet and exercise, but here we'll deal with the problem of toxic emotions. This is extremely important, because abundant evidence demonstrates that emotions play a significant role in the incidence of heart attacks. More attacks, for example, occur early weekday mornings than at any other time. This is not because of an unhealthy diet or a lack of exercise. It's an emotional problem: people literally don't have the heart to go to work.

I recall a sensitive and creative man in his sixties who worked in a fast-growing segment of the publishing industry in the Midwest. He was a talented writer who had received a prestigious prize for poetry during his college years. Though he had played a key role in the company's beginnings, he was later supplanted by younger colleagues. I have no doubt that cynicism and despair took root in his heart as he watched the changing company pass him by. One day he was found dead at the wheel of his car in the company parking lot. The engine was still running. The cause of death was attributed to a heart attack, and it was nine on a Monday morning.

Although negative emotions can literally be deadly, there are many ways to prevent them from taking root in your consciousness. By implementing the seven steps outlined below, you can help your system metabolize and release emotional toxins.

1. Identify the emotion. What are you really feeling? Is it anger, sadness, hurt, betrayal, or some other toxic emotion? Try to define it as clearly as possible.

2. Be mindful of the physical sensations in your body. Negative feelings express themselves not only as thoughts but as actual pain in the body. It may be a headache, muscle stiffness, or chest pains that prefigure a heart attack.

3. Take responsibility for what you're experiencing, and recognize that you have a choice in the matter. You can't always control the circumstances of your life, but you can always control your responses.

4. Express what you're feeling in private. You may want to do this in writing, or even out loud. Do you believe that someone has injured or offended you? If so, imagine that you're speaking directly to that person. What would you say to convey exactly how you feel? What would you write in a letter to that person?

5. Let go of the emotion through some personal ritual. Physical exercise is often useful for this, especially when combined with the Ayurvedic breathing techniques described in chapter 8.

6. Share what you're feeling with another person, but don't undertake this until you feel calm and composed. You should be able to share your feelings without ascribing blame to anyone, and without looking for pity.

7. Celebrate and rejuvenate! Reward yourself for taking control of the situation in ways that are best for physical and emotional health.

5

RISK FACTORS IN

CORONARY HEART DISEASE

A number of well-documented risk factors are associated with coronary heart disease, and each deserves to be discussed in some detail. It's important to remember, however, that a great deal remains to be learned about the causes of CHD and other forms of heart disease. This is especially true because so many heart attacks occur in people who have no known risk factors at all.

Moreover, the identified risk factors are always subject to change. The issue of gender is a case in point. Men have long been considered much more likely than women to develop coronary heart disease, but recently this view has been questioned. It now appears that, in women past age sixty-five, heart disease is much more common than has previously been recognized, and as a result the medical profession has been criticized for failure to sufficiently emphasize heart disease as a factor in women's health. While there is truth to these new findings, data from the National Health Examination Survey indicates that the death rate from heart disease is five times higher in Caucasian men than in Caucasian women in the United States—except for women with high blood pressure, high cholesterol, diabetes, or premature menopause. When we realize that these exceptions constitute a significant number of women, the ambiguities inherent in the risk factors begin to become apparent. At the end of this chapter we will discuss some of the aspects of heart disease unique in women.

Another area that has come under question recently is that of the connection between cholesterol and heart disease. While high cholesterol levels do correlate with heart disease, some scientists now believe that an amino acid in the blood called homocysteine may be a more fundamental cause of the arterial injuries that lead to CHD.

While retaining an awareness of the limits of the risk factor approach, we will discuss six issues in this section that seem to have an important bearing on the development of coronary heart disease. Statistically, a person with at least of one of these factors is more likely to develop coronary heart disease, and to develop it sooner, than a person with none. The presence of more than one risk factor significantly accelerates the process.

The risk factors we will consider are:

1. Cigarette smoking
2. Hypertension
3. Obesity
4. Cholesterol
5. Family history
6. Homocysteine

CIGARETTE SMOKING

Research has established many strong links between smoking and the development of coronary heart disease. For example, with each puff of a cigarette, a smoker inhales a small amount of carbon monoxide, the same deadly gas found in automobile exhaust. The presence of this gas in the blood reduces the amount of oxygen in the bloodstream; this makes the arterial walls more vulnerable to the irritations that are the first phase of coronary heart disease. But carbon monoxide is by no means the only harmful ingredient in cigarette smoke. There are roughly four thousand such substances, whose effects include elevated blood pressure, reduced amounts of HDL ("good" cholesterol), and increased risk of clots forming within blood vessels. In fact, the dangers of cigarette smoking have become so well known that it seems unnecessary to enumerate them here. The statistical bottom line is that cigarette smokers have at least double the risk of developing coronary heart disease as nonsmokers, and the risk grows in proportion to the number of cigarettes smoked each day.

Smoking is unique among the cardiac risk factors because, in theory at least, it can be eliminated immediately. You may have smoked two packs a day for twenty years, but you can choose to become a nonsmoker right now. Moreover, a person who stops smoking cigarettes can quickly reverse the physiological effects, and even a longtime cigarette user may reach the risk level of a nonsmoker within one year of quitting. Indeed, the dividends for giving up this habit can be great.

Because of the well-known dangers of cigarette smoking, many doctors categorically urge their patients to stop at once, and it is difficult to find fault with this advice. But mind/body medicine teaches us to consider the emotional and even the spiritual aspects of any important lifestyle change. If we don't, there are sometimes unintended consequences.

For longtime smokers, cigarettes are a source of a particular kind of pleasure, and there's even a meditative aspect to smoking for many people. Because cigarettes are prohibited in many workplaces, smokers are forced to take a break from their routines, get up from their desks, and spend a few minutes alone or in conversation with other smokers. These are positive experiences for them, and it's even likely they reduce the high levels of stress that are a factor in heart disease. It's unfortunate that when an office worker gives up smoking, he or she also loses the incentive to step outside for a while and do something enjoyable.

In my book *Overcoming Addiction,* I suggest that we as human beings have a basic need for intense pleasure—for a feeling that lifts us above the pains and concerns of everyday life to experience pure joy. I use the word *ecstasy* to refer to that transcendent experience. For many people, however, true ecstasy has become unavailable, and they find themselves turning to substitutes. I believe all forms of addiction, including smoking, are expressions of this thwarted search for true ecstasy. Since addictions are rooted in a deep human need, interventions should be carefully considered. It is not enough to say "Why don't you just quit?" to a person for whom smoking is deeply pleasurable. Although suddenly stopping may work for some people, it is important to respect the needs of those for whom it does not. And although smoking is a secondary form of pleasure, and a poor substitute for true joy, we should be aware that sudden withdrawal from smoking can be a profound shock to the system.

When a person continues to smoke, there can be negative effects from frequent reports of the dangers of smoking. Guilt, fear, and a sense that you can't control your own impulses all afflict the addicted smoker—and these only add to the destructive effects of smoking itself. By pointing this out, I certainly don't mean to suggest that smoking is a healthy activity, or that a smoker should not give up the habit, or that the public should not be made aware of the dangers of tobacco. But I know from my own experience that the pleasures of smoking are very real, and that they can be very difficult to give up unless the problem is addressed at a fundamental level. For the great majority of people, it's not enough simply to want to quit or to be told to quit by a doctor—and in some cases it's not healthy to quit if the change is made too abruptly.

Severe anxiety, the development of substitute addictions, and especially weight gain are frequent side effects of sudden withdrawal from smoking. After years of smoking, the actual pleasure of the act for smokers has often worn off, and lighting a cigarette becomes a "habit" in the true sense of the word.

From an Ayurvedic point of view, smoking is a Vata-related activity. It is something that most people do on impulse, as an attempt to reduce anxiety or as a way of displacing excess energy. Often a smoker lights up a cigarette in response to certain definite cues, which have become so well established that the individual may not even be aware of them.

I believe that understanding this unconscious process of cigarette smoking holds the key to breaking the habit. It's a matter of focusing your attention on the activity, without relying on any form of fear-based motivation. By becoming mindfully aware of the signals that trigger the smoking impulse, you can empower yourself to break the chain of stimulus and response. Loss of awareness leads us to act in ways that run counter to the deeper intelligence within us. So it is not surprising that by putting our full awareness on our smoking habit, we can tune in to what we really want, instead of what we mistakenly think we need.

Putting this into action is surprisingly simple. Don't worry about how much you're smoking. Don't make a hard and fast determination to quit. Both these approaches only create more of the stress that cigarettes are an attempt to get away from. Instead, smoke as much as you want, but when you do, be sure you really want to smoke. Don't respond unconsciously to hidden cues.

The five steps that follow will clarify this approach to breaking the smoking habit.

1. Take a day or two to become aware of the cues that trigger your smoking impulse. Many people reflexively light up a cigarette after a meal or with a cup of coffee. Others smoke while driving or talking on the phone. Whenever you give yourself over to an activity without any conscious attention, the Vata side of your nature is allowed to become dominant by default. So the first step in breaking the smoking habit involves replacing automatic impulse with conscious intention.

2. Stop for a moment whenever you find yourself lighting a cigarette. Ask yourself why you're smoking at this moment in time. Is it simply a reflex that accompanies another activity, or do you really want the cigarette for its own sake? If you find that you're smoking impulsively, put the cigarette out until you genuinely feel a desire for it.

3. When you really want a cigarette, focus on the activity of smoking without any intervening distractions. Find a quiet spot where you can be alone while you smoke.

4. While you're smoking the cigarette, direct your attention to the sensations you experience. How does the smoke taste in your mouth? What does it feel like in your lungs? Are there sensations elsewhere in your body as you inhale and exhale? Instead of just letting the cigarette "smoke itself," make yourself aware of what smoking really feels like.

5. When you're finished with the cigarette, record the time and the location in a small notebook that will be your smoking diary. Also note down what you felt and thought as you smoked. Make a similar note whenever you have a cigarette.

By following these five steps, you'll replace unconscious smoking behavior with mindful attention to what you're doing. This is major progress toward cutting down on cigarettes, and toward eventually breaking the habit entirely.

HYPERTENSION (HIGH BLOOD PRESSURE)

We've taken note of the heart's emotional and spiritual meaning in our lives, but at the simplest level the heart still works as a pump, whose contractions provide the pressure that causes blood to circulate throughout the body. However, when this pressure gets too high, dangerous and even life-threatening conditions can result. Hypertension, the medical term for high blood pressure, can threaten not only the coronary arteries but also the brain, the eyes, and the kidneys. Even more ominously, hypertension can go completely undetected until serious damage has been done. More than half of all Americans over age sixty have high blood pressure, and the percentage continues to rise with age.

Blood pressure can be thought of as a load that the heart muscle must lift with every beat. High blood pressure causes the heart to work harder. The heart is designed to function like a long-distance runner; a healthy heart is tough, lean, and efficient. Hypertension forces the heart to play the role of a weight lifter. Like a weight lifter's biceps, the heart muscle grows larger, but over time it also becomes less efficient in its designated task of pumping blood. If a marathon runner is forced to train while carrying a heavy weight, his body might initially gain mass in an attempt to deal with the problem. But gradually the runner's posture will deteriorate, his stride will shorten, and he'll simply become worn out. In this way hypertension causes long-term weakening of the heart muscle, and often the result is the life-threatening condition known as congestive heart failure. Hypertension can also injure the walls of the coronary arteries, creating the basis for coronary heart disease.

Although taking blood pressure is a standard part of routine physical examinations, few people really understand the pair of numbers that is generated when a physician inflates and deflates a band around their arms. In a typical blood pressure reading of, say, 110/70, the first number is called the systolic pressure and refers to the pressure in the arteries when the heart is contracting. The second number, called the diastolic pressure, measures the pressure when the heart muscle is relaxed between contractions. In adults, a systolic/diastolic reading below 140/90 is considered in normal range; on the other end of the scale, readings above 160/110 indicate severe hypertension.

This may seem simple enough, but in an individual patient the evaluation of blood pressure can become quite complex. Wide variations can occur from moment to moment. The stress of being in a doctor's office, the aftereffects of recent exercise, and even the position you're sitting in can skew the reading. In fact, more than one-third of patients who show high blood pressure on a single reading are in the normal range when the test is performed again. Clearly, a diagnosis of hypertension requires careful and repeated evaluations.

The causes of high blood pressure may vary widely from patient to patient. Sometimes the causes seem obvious: massive obesity, for example, or heavy alcohol use, or a sedentary lifestyle. Yet hypertension may also afflict individuals who display none of these characteristics. Severe high blood pressure seems to run in families, but individual family members may be entirely unaffected.

Pharmaceutical companies have created dozens of drugs for hypertension, and more are always on the way. Many patients, particularly among the elderly, take several of these medications at once, as well as other drugs to control side effects. If your physician prescribes high blood pressure medications, I suggest that you ask for a thorough explanation of how the drug works, the potential risks and benefits, and the side effects to be expected, as well as how it may interact with any other medications you may be taking.

Interventions such as healthy diet, appropriate exercise, and daily meditation are every bit as important as drugs in treating high blood pressure. In fact, the National Institutes of Health has recognized the power of meditation to reduce stress, and recommends meditation instead of medication for cases of mild hypertension. If a careful physical exam has revealed that you're suffering from hypertension, the lifestyle changes described in part 2 of this book can bring very significant benefits.

OBESITY

Massively obese people are at higher risk for many illnesses, including cancer, diabetes, and coronary heart disease. When overweight is less than extreme, however, the situation becomes much more complex with regard to heart disease. Because it is difficult to arrive at an objective standard for what an individual should weigh at a given age and height, two people with the same reading on a scale can be at very different risk levels. A muscular athlete may weigh much more than a sedentary individual of the same height, but this weight in no way reflects their relative risk for heart trouble.

Evidence supports the theory that the distribution of weight around the body may be more important in heart disease than the actual number of pounds. Men, for example, tend to accumulate fat above the waist, in the abdomen and the chest. This reflects a greater risk of heart problems than the typical female pattern of fat accumulation in the hips and thighs.

There is probably no larger enterprise in America than the weight-control industry. There is also no fatter population in the world than the United States, and it's getting fatter all the time. But as with smoking and hypertension, sudden, extreme measures to lose weight can be counterproductive and even dangerous. This is especially true when, as often happens, an individual's weight fluctuates dramatically as he or she goes on and off various diets. In general, the healthiest approaches to weight control are those that emphasize the pleasures of food and eating while minimizing the fear and anxiety associated with overweight. This topic is covered in more detail in part 2, as well as in my book *Perfect Weight.*

CHOLESTEROL

Cholesterol is a type of fat known as a lipid. It is manufactured naturally by the body, but diet can account for a great deal of additional cholesterol. For the past twenty years, the term "high cholesterol" has become almost synonymous with "heart attack." According to the Multiple Risk Factor Intervention Trial, an extremely authoritative long-term investigation of the causes of heart disease, men between the ages of 35 and 57 whose total cholesterol measured 300 milligrams per deciliter were four times more likely to die of coronary heart disease within six years than men whose cholesterol level was under 180 milligrams per deciliter (mg/dl).

The message is clear: get your blood cholesterol as low as possible, and keep it there. It's hard to argue that this is poor advice, but a closer look at cholesterol reveals some important nuances.

Blood is mostly water. Ideally, it's a thin, oxygen-rich solution that passes smoothly through the body's veins and arteries. The presence of fats and oils in the blood makes blood thicker and heavier, so the heart must work harder at circulation. But the significance of cholesterol goes beyond simply elevating the density of blood. When arterial walls have been irritated or damaged, the type of cholesterol known as low-density lipoprotein (LDL) tends to accumulate at the site of the injury. Eventually this accumulation develops into a thick plaque, narrowing the artery and setting the stage for a heart attack. The second kind of cholesterol is high-density lipoprotein (HDL)—the so-called good cholesterol. It can have the opposite effect, actually working to eliminate arterial blockages. Therefore the ratio of "bad" to "good" cholesterol in the blood is a very important figure.

For our purposes two important points should be made regarding cholesterol. First, you can reduce the cholesterol content of your blood by making changes in your diet. Practical suggestions for accomplishing this are provided later in this book, but the impact of dietary changes on cholesterol is directly related to the extent of the changes themselves.

Second, if you are intent on radically lowering your cholesterol count, you will most likely need to make radical changes beyond what you eat. As we discussed in regard to smoking, such radical changes will have an effect on all areas of your life, not just the walls of your arteries. Some changes may be beneficial and others less so, but in a holistic approach to health all these changes deserve your attention. You may lengthen your life by reducing your cholesterol, but this benefit is undermined if your pleasure in living is also reduced. On the other hand, if you view a low cholesterol count not as an absolute value in itself, but as an indicator that you're living the way you really want to live, then you've helped your heart in a real way.

FAMILY HISTORY

The role of heredity in coronary heart disease is fraught with misunderstandings. This much seems clear: if your parents or other close relatives died of a heart attack before the age of fifty, your risk of developing coronary artery disease is statistically greater than a person with no family history. This seems to be true even when other risk factors that were accepted in previous generations, such as smoking, have been eliminated.

More specifically, people whose families show a tendency toward extremely high cholesterol levels (of 300 mg/dl and above) are at greater risk for early onset of heart disease.

The notion that your family history predisposes you to a heart attack, however, contains risks that may be greater than the genetic ones. No one should feel "fated" to have a heart attack. In the United States, approximately 1 in 500 deaths is attributable to the apparently inherited high cholesterol levels referred to above—but the percentage of deaths caused by coronary disease as a whole is many orders of magnitude larger. Compared to illnesses in which family plays a truly important role—cystic fibrosis, for example—the influence of heredity on heart disease is insignificant. In any event, focusing on the past, which is out of our control, can only distract our attention from beneficial activities which are much more important: diet, exercise, and learning to bring true happiness into our lives.

HOMOCYSTEINE

The onset of coronary heart disease is often attributed to injuries sustained by the coronary arteries. At the site of an arterial injury, cholesterol and blood platelets gather, forming the plaque that narrows the lining of the artery causing blockages of blood flow to the heart.

As we have discussed, smoking and hypertension are two causes of arterial damage. Another culprit is a toxic amino acid derived from a diet high in animal protein, called homocysteine. It is likely that you will hear more and more about homocysteine and its role in heart disease in the future, as some researchers believe it may turn out to be an even more important factor than cholesterol in determining if you are at risk.

In 1969, Dr. Kilmer McCully of Harvard first theorized that

homocysteine might play a key role in the development of heart disease. His theory had its roots in two cases he had seen in his role as a pathologist, when he observed a strange phenomenon in two young children who had a rare disease called homocystinuria. This disease, which results in an abnormally high blood level of homocysteine, led to the death of both children from severe arteriosclerosis. McCully then wondered if there might be a link between homocysteine and heart disease. At the time, the cholesterol theory of heart disease was receiving much attention, and McCully could not get the funding he needed to continue his research. Today, however, it is believed that his theory has great validity.

In a long-running study of almost 15,000 healthy doctors, it was determined that high levels of homocysteine correlate with a three-fold increase in risk of heart attack. Other research has shown that in young women high homocysteine doubles the risk of heart attack. In still another study, high blood homocysteine levels were seen in almost one-third of adults age sixty-seven or older.

The homocysteine theory fits in well with other known factors in heart disease. For example, the B vitamins help to reduce levels of homocysteine in the blood. Interestingly, the rise in heart disease in women coincides with the use of the birth control pill, which lowers B_6 levels. Smoking, another risk factor for heart disease, also lowers B_6. Folic acid, one of the B-complex vitamins, is often deficient in the American diet. A diet high in meat protein, eggs, or cheese, and low in green leafy vegetables and whole grains, may result in B-vitamin deficiencies and high levels of homocysteine.

Fortunately, it is believed that homocysteine levels can be brought down to safe levels quite easily through dietary changes and vitamin supplements.

HEART DISEASE IN WOMEN: SPECIAL ISSUES

While many women may secretly worry that their husband will drop dead of a heart attack while fighting traffic, stressing out at work, or exerting himself during sex, few women seem to believe that they themselves will die of a heart attack. That heart disease is a male problem is a strange myth indeed, and a potentially dangerous one for women who are genuinely at risk. In fact, almost half of Americans who die from heart disease each year are women. Approximately 250,000 women will die of coronary artery disease this year, making it the most common cause of death among American women.

Some women have a significantly higher risk than others for succumbing to heart disease. This higher-risk group includes women who are postmenopausal, diabetic, smokers, both users of birth control and smokers, and overweight.

Today, women with heart disease or women who are at risk for heart disease are at a disadvantage with regard to its diagnosis and treatment. Much of this can be attributed to the fact that in the past most research on heart disease was devoted to studying men. Underdiagnosis of heart disease in women is all too common, as both physicians and women fail to make the connection between their symptoms and heart disease. Also, some cardiac diagnostic tests, such as the stress test, were designed using male subjects. When women take these tests, their results are often difficult to interpret. If diagnosed properly, the current treatments for heart disease, such as coronary bypass surgery, are less effective in women. And women seem to do less well socially and psychologically after suffering a heart attack or receiving treatment for coronary artery disease. This may explain why the mortality rate within two months of a first heart attack is twice as high in women as in men. Women are also three times more likely to have another heart attack in the same year. This may stem from the fact that women who have heart attacks are usually older than men, so their overall health is likely to be less good.

As we have previously discussed, awareness is one of the main pathways to healing. Women as well as men need to be aware of the risk factors and symptoms of heart disease so they can act in ways that protect their hearts, as well as acknowledge and attend to any problems that may arise.

Fear of coronary heart disease motivates many people to modify their lifestyle, but I would like to emphasize, in ending this section, that fear-motivated behavior cannot be successful in the long run. Fear may cause you to eat a salad instead of a hamburger, it may impel you to turn off the television and take a walk around the block—but fear itself has its own biological effects, and they are decidedly unhealthy. If fear of a high cholesterol count turns every meal into an occasion for anxiety, you would do better simply to forget about monitoring your cholesterol and eat whatever you really enjoy.

We cannot separate the end results of an action from its beginnings. We cannot evaluate the physiological benefits of a lifestyle change without considering its emotional and spiritual origins. The key to eliminating risk factors lies in joyful acceptance of the fact that Nature intends us to be well. Good health, therefore, is not an act of will. It is simply a matter of recognizing and following our true natural inclinations.

PART TWO

REVERSING CORONARY HEART DISEASE

CURRENT STRATEGIES

IN WESTERN MEDICINE

Coronary heart disease takes a number of different forms. In some people the disease appears suddenly and dramatically, while in others it proceeds gradually along a predictable course. In this chapter, we will review five forms of CHD, along with a brief consideration of current mainstream approaches to treatment.

The four CHD categories are: silent ischemia; stable angina pectoris; unstable angina pectoris; and heart attack (myocardial infarction).

SILENT ISCHEMIA

Ischemia is a Latinate word meaning blockage or restraint of blood circulation, such as occurs within the coronary arteries when they are afflicted by CHD. Silent ischemia refers to blockage that does not produce any manifest symptoms.

Often this condition is discovered only by a stress test or an electrocardiogram administered during a routine physical exam. Since there are no symptoms to treat in silent ischemia, the response options of conventional medicine are limited. It isn't even clear that the silent ischemia revealed through diagnostic tests is an accurate predictor of more severe problems in the future. Some patients choose to undergo further examination, while others are simply cautioned to be on the lookout for further symptoms and are sent on their way.

There are no nerve endings inside coronary arteries to alert us of damage or blockages. Even if chest pain does appear, the pain threshold of the individual or other masking symptoms may allow the problem to remain hidden. Not infrequently silent ischemia can do great damage with no awareness on the part of the patient. Severe heart attacks can occur with no pain whatsoever, and the damage to the heart muscle may only be discovered much later. Data from the long-term Framingham heart study showed that approximately 15 percent of all heart attacks were "silent," and an equal number of attacks were wrongly perceived as indigestion or some other problem. In many cases, of course, we don't know how a heart attack has been perceived, because it is fatal.

STABLE ANGINA PECTORIS:
PRUDENCE AND PILLS

Angina pectoris means, quite simply, "pain in the chest." Frequently, this pain is brought on by blockage of the coronary arteries. If pain appears under a predictable set of circumstances, and if it remains consistent rather than growing more severe with each appearance, the condition is referred to as stable angina pectoris.

For example, a businessman who spends much of the day sitting down may not experience any discomfort during his regular routine. But whenever he tries to play soccer with his children, he suffers pain in his chest. The blood flow through his partially blocked arteries is adequate for his everyday needs, but when vigorous exercise increases the heart muscle's demand for oxygen, there is not enough blood to meet the demand.

The symptoms of stable angina can often be avoided by prudence on the part of the patient. If the businessman plays cards with his children instead of soccer, he won't have chest pains. The condition of his coronary arteries won't improve unless he adopts a healthier lifestyle, but years may go by before his symptoms worsen.

A large number of medications are frequently prescribed for stable angina pectoris. Nitroglycerin, for example, in the form of a pill, a spray, or a patch, temporarily dilates the coronary arteries and eliminates the pain. Many people with stable angina are advised to take nitroglycerin before beginning any activity that they anticipate will strain the heart. Other commonly prescribed drugs include calcium channel blockers, which reduce the heart's demand for oxygen as well as dilating the arteries, and beta blockers, which slow the heart rate and reduce blood pressure.

In the past decade, aspirin has received a great deal of attention both as a preventive agent for first heart attacks and for maintaining cardiac health in recovering heart attack patients. In one important study involving more than 20,000 participants over a period of four years, subjects who took half an aspirin tablet each day suffered 40 percent fewer heart attacks than a control group. But despite its demonstrated effectiveness, there are drawbacks to aspirin therapy. While the drug seems to lower the risk of heart attacks, it may raise the risk of strokes. In significant numbers of people, aspirin can also irritate the digestive system and increase vulnerability to ulcers. Lastly, the correct dosage for aspirin therapy has never been established.

UNSTABLE ANGINA PECTORIS

Unstable angina is characterized by worsening, increasingly unpredictable chest pain. Often it is unclear why the chest pain becomes turbulent—growing stronger, then receding, then intensifying again—but this always indicates a fragile situation. Frequently the cause is a blood clot forming in a coronary artery that is already partially blocked. In any event, most physicians usually order hospitalization. Medications begin at once, and your cardiologist will consider such procedures as thallium scan, angiography, angioplasty, and bypass surgery.

Thallium Scan

In a *thallium scan,* a small amount of radioactive material is injected into the bloodstream. As this material enters the coronary arteries, sensitive instruments are used to monitor its spread. Ideally, a thallium scan is performed in conjunction with exercise, but this is not always possible. The scan provides a picture of the effect of blockages on the heart muscle, though not of the blockages themselves.

Angiography

Angiograms are almost always recommended when a patient is hospitalized for unstable angina in order to determine the size, position, and degree of danger posed by coronary artery blockages. An angiogram is a type of X ray. A special contrast dye is injected into the coronary arteries through a long, thin tube called a catheter, which is threaded toward the heart through a blood vessel. As the contrast dye enters various areas of the heart, X rays are taken to assess the extent of CHD. Although angiography is common and the statistical risks are small, it is a major procedure. It requires a period of rest in a recovery room, and patients are usually advised to stay off their feet for six to eight hours afterward.

Angiography is an extremely useful tool in the evaluation of coronary heart disease, but it has its drawbacks and limitations. Hundreds of thousands of angiograms are performed every year, at a cost of millions of dollars, and it is questionable whether all these procedures are necessary. Quite often angiography is presented to patients as part of a continuum leading to angioplasty and/or bypass surgery, as if there were no noninvasive treatment options. Today, the implied purpose of angiography is to determine whether an angioplasty or a bypass is indicated—and in a large number of cases it turns out that these invasive procedures are indeed deemed necessary.

It's worth noting, however, that an angiogram by no means provides an infallible or complete picture of the state of CHD. Although it relies on expensive, sophisticated equipment and highly trained medical professionals, there can be significant differences of opinion in interpreting the test results. One physician may feel that an artery is much more severely blocked than it appears to another doctor. In addition, angiography is much more effective in disclosing bumps in the arteries than more uniform buildups of plaque along the arterial walls. This could cause the degree of generalized arterial narrowing to be underestimated.

Setting aside the question of reliability, every heart patient should be wary of tacit suggestions that an angiogram is simply a preliminary to angioplasty or bypass surgery. There are alternatives to such interventions, including changes in diet, exercise, and other approaches discussed later in this book. The possible usefulness of these alternative methods for reversing coronary heart disease deserves to be thoroughly explored before turning to invasive procedures.

Angioplasty

Angioplasty is virtually always used with angiography to create a sort of one-two punch against coronary heart disease. Once the location of an arterial blockage has been located by angiogram, the angioplasty catheter is inserted into a blood vessel and threaded directly into the coronary artery. When the point of the blockage is reached, the balloon at the tip of the catheter is inflated, forcing the blockage back into the arterial wall and clearing the artery for increased blood flow. In about one-third of all cases, blockages return within a year and the procedure must be repeated. Currently, other forms of catheterization are being introduced that use rotating disks or lasers instead of balloons.

Although several hundred thousand angioplasties are performed each year, this intervention is not appropriate for every case of coronary artery disease. The ideal candidate has a well-functioning heart, particularly in the crucial area of the left ventricle, with only a few blockages in the coronary arteries. Of course, this type of patient is also a good candidate for other noninvasive forms of treatment. Although the death rate for patients who have undergone angioplasty is low (less than 1 percent), the death rate for these individuals would probably have remained low even if they had not undergone the procedure.

Bypass Surgery

Coronary bypass surgery involves the creation of a "detour" around blocked areas of the coronary arteries. It is recommended when one or more coronary arteries has become severely impaired and angioplasty has been deemed inappropriate. During the surgery, heart and lung functions are temporarily taken over by a machine while the surgeon grafts bypasses onto the coronary arteries using segments of veins taken from the legs. In an alternative procedure, branches of arteries already present in the heart, known as the internal mammary arteries, are "rewired" and there is no need for the removal of veins from elsewhere in the body. As with angioplasty, hundreds of thousands of bypass surgeries are performed each year. When multiple bypasses are necessary, the operation can last as long as eight hours and can cost more than $100,000.

The goals of bypass surgery are, first, to relieve the imminent danger of a potentially fatal heart attack and, second, to improve the quality of life in patients who have become severely debilitated by unstable angina. These goals are achieved in a large majority of cases. However, just as a detour around an impassable stretch of highway does not repair the damaged road, bypass surgery does not affect the underlying causes of coronary artery blockages. Within ten years of their bypass operations, as many as 40 percent of all patients are again suffering from coronary heart disease; sometimes new blockages form in the bypasses themselves. No one should think of bypass surgery as a long-term solution to a heart problem. At best, the operation buys time for a patient to make the crucial lifestyle changes that eliminate the causes as well as the effects of CHD.

HEART ATTACK

When a coronary artery has become completely blocked, the area of the heart muscle nourished by that artery is denied oxygen, and the tissue quickly becomes necrotic; it dies. Depending on the size and location of the affected area, heart function can be impaired or completely destroyed. This is what happens during a heart attack. *Myocardial infarction* is the medical term: the myocardium is the heart muscle, and an infarction is an area of tissue damaged by oxygen deprivation.

Most heart attacks occur when a clot becomes lodged in an already narrowed coronary artery and cuts off the flow of blood completely. The patient typically experiences a prolonged, painful sensation of pressure in the chest, often accompanied by sharp, shooting pain in the left shoulder, the left arm, and the jaw. There may be nausea, sweating, and shortness of breath. Despite the dramatic nature of these symptoms, heart attack victims sometimes deny or fail to recognize what's happening. For this reason, 60 percent of people who die from a first heart attack succumb within one hour of symptom onset, and before seeking any medical help.

Although a heart attack can strike suddenly, Ayurveda teaches that every illness carries warning signals that must be heeded if the progress of the disease is to be stopped and reversed. The long-term warning signals of coronary heart disease include being overweight, persistent feelings of hostility, angina, and other topics we've discussed. In the short term, heart attack victims often feel exhausted, hopeless, or depressed in the days before the event. But no warning is sufficient if a person's *awareness* has become closed off to the body's internal signals.

You don't need a stethoscope to listen to your heart. Starting today, make a conscious decision to focus awareness on your heart and on the core issues in your life that it symbolizes. In the next chapter you'll learn techniques to help you do exactly that.

7

MEDITATION

Ayurveda offers many practical methods for creating and preserving health, but I believe that meditation is by far the most powerful and the most important. Like the heart, which is of such great significance both physically and spiritually, meditation engages us at all levels of our being, transcending distinctions between body, mind, and spirit.

Though meditation is often portrayed as a relaxation technique, this an incomplete picture of its purpose in the Ayurvedic tradition. Meditation is indeed intended to discover silence in the mind, but making this discovery is not really the same thing as simply relaxing. The ancient sages of India were already quite relaxed by the time they began to meditate. Their intention was something much more profound. Through the practice of meditation—whether it's mindfulness meditation, primordial sound meditation using a mantra, or the heart sutra meditation—you can create an internal reference

point of Spirit rather than ego. You can enter the silent spaces
between your thoughts, the gap in which ego-based concerns
disappear and the thinker, the process of thinking, and the
object of thought are revealed as one.

This may sound a bit abstract and philosophical, but there
is no doubt that meditation can have tangible benefits for the
heart. In the late 1970s, a study done in Israel found that twice-
daily meditation brought about an average 30-point drop in
cholesterol levels among a group of subjects whose previous
readings had been above 255—and meditation was also effective with subjects whose initial readings had been in a more
normal range. This improvement would be difficult to match
by any program of diet or exercise. Indeed, my personal belief
is that your mental and emotional state is more important in
lowering or exacerbating cholesterol levels than any other factor. By allowing us to enter a state of restful alertness in our
minds, meditation literally transforms the chemistry of our
bodies.

MINDFULNESS MEDITATION

This is one of the easiest and most accessible forms of meditation, but it is also an effective and powerful technique. By
focusing your awareness on your breathing, mindfulness meditation can quiet the everyday static of your thoughts. This, in
turn, facilitates healing in the heart and throughout the body.

Practice this meditation technique twice each day, in the
morning and in the early evening, for 20 to 30 minutes per session. Find a quiet, pleasant space for yourself where you won't
be disturbed, and follow these seven steps:

1. Close your eyes. (10 seconds)
2. Gently focus awareness on your breathing. As you inhale and exhale, observe your breath. (30 seconds)

3. Remain aware of your breathing, without trying to alter it in anyway. (15 seconds)

4. As you observe your breath, it may vary in speed, rhythm, or depth. It may even seem to stop for a time. Without resisting, calmly observe these changes. (1 minute)

5. At the beginning of the session, your attention may drift to a thought passing through your mind, to a physical sensation in your body, or to some other distraction. If you notice that you are not observing your breath, gently refocus your attention. (1 minute)

6. Relinquish any expectations you may have during the practice of this technique. If you find yourself being drawn to a particular feeling, mood, or expectation, treat this as you would any other thought. Gently return your awareness to your breath. (20 to 30 minutes)

7. Open your eyes slowly, returning your attention to the sights and sounds around you.

You can extend this technique by gradually shifting your awareness from your breathing to your heart. To do this, feel the stream of your breath flowing into the center of your chest as you inhale. Think of your heart as an empty space that is being filled with your breath. Of course, this is very much like what actually happens when blood passing through your lungs acquires oxygen and flows back into your heart.

When you've allowed your attention to remain on your heart for several minutes, slowly open your eyes as in normal breathing meditation.

PRIMORDIAL SOUND MEDITATION

Primordial sounds are natural vibrations that structure the universe. Just as plants grow from seeds, entire languages spring from these basic syllables. We hear sounds everywhere in Nature, in wind blowing through trees, in waves crashing against rocks. Ayurveda teaches that listening to primordial sounds can restore our sense of connection to the whole of creation, and enliven the healing energy within us.

Primordial Sound Meditation uses the root sounds of the Sanskrit alphabet to create mantras. These sounds have no meaning in normal speech. Because they are free of the associations that accompany everyday words, primordial sounds temporarily interrupt the otherwise continuous flow of our thoughts. With practice, Primordial Sound Meditation can give you access to a profound level of silence and healing.

At The Chopra Center for Well Being and at seminars organized by the center, Primordial Sound Meditation is taught by trained instructors. Information is provided at the end of this book.

BRAIN WAVE AND HEART WAVE COHERENCE

In addition to its many other remarkable capabilities, the human body is also a generator of electromagnetic energy. The preponderance of this energy originates in the brain and in the sinoatrial node of the heart, which was described in chapter 2. The heart's electrical energy, however, is far stronger than that of the brain—as much as 40 to 60 times stronger. But the raw strength of the energy is less significant than a quality known as *coherence*.

A high level of brain wave coherence, for example, is present if the pattern of brain waves at a given frequency is constant, when measured by electrodes at various areas of the scalp. Most people have rather low levels of brain wave coherence. The turbulence of their internal dialogue is such that the wave at one location is clearly out of synch with the others. High brain wave coherence, on the other hand, correlates with strong learning ability, memory, attention span, creativity, and even healing.

Similarly, the electromagnetic waves of the heart can be measured for their coherence. The electrical energy originating in the sinoatrial node may be chaotic and incoherent when measured at various locations on the organ—or a high degree of regularity and synchronization may be present, which is characteristic of a healthy heart.

To a certain extent, the electromagnetic activities of the heart and the brain exist independently. A human heart can be completely removed from the body and, if placed in a hospitable medium and supplied with the proper nutrients, will continue to beat indefinitely: The heart does not need the brain as a power source. High levels of brain wave coherence can definitely influence the electrical activity of the heart, however, so that the flow of energy becomes synchronized in the two organs and throughout the body. This can have profound benefits for cardiac health.

Meditation is an extremely effective way of increasing brain wave coherence, and thus of healing the heart. Research at the Institute of HeartMath, in Boulder Creek, California, has shown that meditative states of mind can help stabilize the heart's electromagnetic field. Such "heartfelt" emotions as joy, appreciation, and love have a similar effect. By kindling these feelings and drawing on their power, the heart sutra meditation described below allows your mind to directly and positively influence your heart.

HEART SUTRA

The Sanskrit word *sutra* is related to such English words as "suture," "stitch," and "ligature," which are themselves the origins of the word *religion,* which literally means "to stitch" or "to tie back." One might say that, through religion, we stitch the self. We repair the soul. We heal the body. These are the purposes of sutra practice, which is an advanced form of meditation.

Mindfulness meditation and Primordial Sound Mediation enable us to reach a level of deep silence. With sutra practice, we bring a faint impulse of intelligence into that stillness. It's as if you were to drop a tiny pebble into a very still pond. A little ripple is created, which radiates in all directions. Sutra meditation introduces a wisp of intention into the stillness of consciousness.

Begin this meditation with 5 to 10 minutes of breathing awareness, then gradually shift your awareness toward your heart. Next, very gently and without any force whatsoever, introduce the intention of *stillness* into your mind and your body. Let the stillness of your thoughts radiate through your physical self like soft ripples in a pond. Feel the stillness bringing your mind and your heat together.

Now let four words enter and pass through your consciousness. These are the sutras—spiritual stitches to mend and strengthen heart, mind, and soul.

The sutras are:

> Peace . . .
> Harmony . . .
> Laughter . . .
> Love . . .

Silently repeat each of these words four times, with a pause of 10 to 15 seconds between each repetition. Each time the word enters your consciousness, feel it rippling out through your body, and even outside your body into the universe beyond. With time, you'll be able to do this while still maintaining a deep stillness of mind and spirit. When you learn to nurture the faint presence of a thought within a profound

inner silence, wave coherence of your heart and your brain is achieved.

Think of meditation being just like any other natural process: You don't try to breathe, you just breathe. Your hair won't try to grow, it just grows. You don't ever try to meditate—you just meditate. At best, it's a spontaneous process. You may even fall asleep while you're meditating. If you do, accept it as completely appropriate. You probably need the rest!

Ayurveda teaches us never to judge the quality of meditation by the meditation itself. It's not like a movie, a game, or a meal. Don't worry about doing it the right or wrong way, because those terms don't apply. Don't look backward and judge your performance. Instead, look forward with joy to the healing effects of meditation on your heart, and on every area of your life.

8

EXERCISE

When you were very young, almost any form of physical exercise was fun. Running and jumping and playing were their own rewards. But as we age, the meaning of exercise also changes: for an athlete, it becomes a medium of competition; for a daily jogger, it is a means of staying in shape; for an overweight, sedentary person, it is something to be avoided. Ayurveda teaches that all forms of exercise—or even refusing to exercise—can serve the same essential purpose of *establishing communication with your body.*

This is not to suggest that watching television all day can do as much for your health as running five miles a day. Rather, it means that both a marathon runner and a couch potato can listen to and learn from the messages their bodies are sending— and if they're wise, they can begin to adjust their activities accordingly. The runner may feel a pain in her heel: this is a message that she should reduce her training mileage. The inactive person may feel sluggish and depressed: his emotional self is shutting down because his physical self is being neglected.

And, of course, both of these people may also receive warning messages from their hearts—in the form of pain, irregular rhythms, or even fainting. Once these two quite different individuals have responded to their internal signals, other, more satisfactory signals will be sent. The open line of communication between mind and body will have served its purpose.

Learning to understand the messages of your body may require a bit of time and focused attention. If you've been leading an inactive life, or if you've grown accustomed to exerting yourself to the limit, you may have lost the ability to understand your body's real language. You may misinterpret anxiety-driven sugar cravings as real hunger, or you may convince yourself that a genuine need for rest is a sign of weakness that ought to be ignored. So before you begin an Ayurvedic exercise program, you should be aware of three principles that hold true regardless of your body type, and that can be easily recognized no matter how out of touch you may have grown from your body's true needs.

1. **Exercise only to 50 percent of your capacity.** This is the point where your breathing begins to be labored, where your motions become less fluid, and where you begin to be aware of strain. With a little practice, you'll be able to recognize this point accurately, and research has shown that perceived levels of exertion can be as accurate as stress tests or heart monitors. As your conditioning improves, your halfway-to-the-limit point will also increase proportionally.

2. **Exercise regularly—every day if possible.** If you're exercising at the right level of intensity and for the proper amount of time, you'll look forward to doing so every day. If you begin to shy away from exercising, it's a sign that you've been working too hard.

3. **Let your breath and perspiration guide you.** If your breathing grows short and you're perspiring heavily, you're putting too much strain on your body. You should always be

able to breathe through your nose while exercising. If you have to breathe through your mouth, cut back.

(CAUTION: **If you have a history of heart disease or have not been physically active for some time, no exercise program should be undertaken before you consult a physician.**)

EXERCISE FOR THE DOSHAS

In order to gain maximum benefit from exercise you should choose activities that balance your particular physiology. If you haven't been exercising regularly, however, it's a good idea to start with a light level of activity regardless of your mind/body type. Once again, consult your health care provider before beginning any exercise program.

• **Vata types** favor light exercises that emphasize balance and stretching, because Vata dosha can easily be thrown out of balance by overexertion. If Vata is your predominant dosha, easy walking, bicycling, yoga, and dance are best suited for you.

• **Pitta types** enjoy challenges, but they also tend to push themselves too hard. Brisk walking, jogging, skiing, bicycling, and swimming are good Pitta activities, but remember to approach them as playful enjoyments rather than intense competitions. An overly competitive frame of mind—even if you're only competing against yourself—can easily give rise to anger and hostility, which are incompatible with cardiac health.

• **Kapha types** require vigorous exercise, and activities that emphasize endurance. Running, bicycling, swimming, weight training, and aerobics are appropriate for Kaphas. Although they're sometimes slow getting started, Kaphas have excellent stamina, and can benefit from the experience of friendly athletic competition. Developing a program of regular physical exercise is an opportunity for Kaphas to break free of their tendencies for prolonged inactivity and unhealthy eating habits, both of which can foster coronary heart disease.

BREATHING

Everyone knows what happens if we stop breathing, so it seems almost comical to emphasize the importance of breathing in exercise. But Ayurveda teaches that breathing is not just a matter of taking air into the lungs. The act of drawing breath has profound significance, both biologically and spiritually.

The Sanskrit word *prana* refers to the vital energy that animates all living things, and breathing is the primary means of bringing that energy into the body. With every breath, you exchange billions of atoms with the universe, which is your extended body. As you inhale, you draw nourishment from the environment, including the oxygen that passes directly from your lungs into your bloodstream. If oxygen is plentiful in your breath and in your blood, your heart and your entire body will benefit. But if your breath is clogged with tobacco smoke or other pollutants, the presence of oxygen diminishes and your overall health suffers. Oxygen-poor blood, for example, is a major cause of irritation to coronary artery walls. This irritation in turn sets the stage for coronary heart disease.

Breathing with awareness, whether during meditation or exercise, is highly beneficial to your overall good health, so take every opportunity to focus on this vital activity. Concentrate on breathing deeply and regularly through your nose, drawing the air in by expanding your diaphragm. Whenever you feel tired or under pressure, breathing with intention and awareness can help both physically and emotionally.

Breathing Exercises

Pranayama is the Ayurvedic science of breath. Through the pranayama breathing exercises described below, you can learn to consciously activate and direct the life force as it enters and becomes part of you. In Western scientific terms, you can increase both the capacity of your lungs and the volume of oxygen that passes into your blood with each breath.

After completing any breathing exercise, take a few moments to rest. Keep your eyes closed, breathe slowly and evenly, and draw your attention inward. Be aware of your body and of the sensations that you're experiencing in any part of it. This rest period is an important part of all pranayama techniques.

• **Ujjayi,** which means "control through expansion" in Sanskrit, is a breathing exercise for cooling the back of your throat. Because it is also an efficient way of bringing oxygen into your lungs and the bloodstream, Ujjayi can be considered the most important pranayama technique for the heart.

> *Begin by whispering "ha." Focus your attention on the point where the breath originates in your throat. Then close your mouth, breathe through your nose, and without vocalizing create this same soft whispering sound, which comes as you breathe from the back of your throat.*
>
> *As you continue to breathe you'll be able to feel air striking the roof of your mouth. Keep the sound smooth and light. Close your eyes and continue to breathe easily for a few breaths. There is no need to force your breath in or out; your breathing should sound like gentle snoring.*

It's best to perform Ujjayi in five cycles over a period of 2 to 3 minutes. Ujjayi helps to expand, lengthen, and deepen your breath. Perhaps most important, it also slows the heart rate, an effect that can be observed using technologies such as fluoroscopy and electrocardiography. Ujjayi has been used by highly trained athletes to reduce fatigue during demanding exercise, as well as cardiac patients who need maximum nourishment from every breath and every heartbeat. Although Ujjayi can be extremely valuable in reversing coronary heart disease, this technique is not appropriate for patients whose hearts beat too slowly or who suffer from arrhythmia.

• **Nadi Shodhana,** which means "channel purification" in Sanskrit, is alternate nostril breathing. By balancing your breath and by focusing your attention on your breathing, this relieves stress and restores physiological balance. It is particularly effective in soothing the effects of unbalanced Vata.

> *To begin, sit in a comfortable chair with your back straight and your feet flat on the floor.*
>
> *Remain quiet for a moment, then gently draw your attention to your breath.*
>
> *Place the thumb of your right hand beside your right nostril and your two middle fingers beside your left nostril.*
>
> *Gently close the right nostril with your thumb, as you slowly exhale through the left nostril.*
>
> *Now inhale easily through the left nostril, then close the left nostril with the two middle fingers and exhale out the right nostril.*
>
> *Now inhale easily through the right nostril. Once again, gently close the right nostril with your thumb, as you slowly exhale through the left nostril.*
>
> *Now inhale easily through the left nostril. Close the left nostril with the two middle fingers and exhale out of the right nostril.*
>
> *Now inhale easily through the right nostril.*

This concludes two cycles of Nadi Shodhana. Notice the pause between each breath, and be sure to keep your breathing long, slow, and refined. Perform three complete cycles of Nadi Shodhana with each nostril over a period of 4 to 5 minutes.

• **Bhrimari,** which means "bumble bee" in Sanskrit, can be used to overcome insomnia and promote the restful sleep essential for a healthy heart.

> *Sit in a comfortable chair with your back straight and your feet flat on the floor.*
> *Take a deep breath, and then make a low humming deep in your throat as you slowly exhale through your nose.*
> *Now inhale again through your nose, and repeat the humming sound as you exhale.*

Perform five cycles of Bhrimari over a period of 2 to 3 minutes.

• **Sitali,** which means "cooling" in Sanskrit, is useful for pacifying the anger and competitiveness that characterizes unbalanced Pitta. Use this technique whenever you're feeling angry and overheated, whether physically or emotionally.

> *Begin by curling your tongue into a tunnel shape, as if you were about to sip water through your tongue.*
> *Exhale through your nose or from the back of your throat as in the Ujjayi breathing exercise.*
> *Create a sipping sound as you inhale—feel the cooling sensation of your breath, and then exhale through your nose.*

Repeat this breathing cycle easily and smoothly for five cycles over 2 to 3 minutes.

• **Kapalabhati,** which means "lustrous head" in Sanskrit, stimulates Kapha and draws invigorating energy into the mind/

body system. It is helpful in overcoming the sedentary lifestyle tendencies that are associated with many cases of coronary heart disease.

> *Sit comfortably on the floor or in a chair with your back straight and your feet flat on the floor.*
> *Begin by exhaling forcefully through your nose, vigorously contracting your diaphragm or belly. Emphasize the exhale as you passively allow the inhale to come in.*
> *Continue to emphasize your exhale as you breathe evenly.*

Perform three cycles of ten breaths each, with a minute of slow, deep breathing between each cycle. Be sure to stop the exercise or reduce the number of repetitions if you feel light-headed or uncomfortable.

YOGA

Earlier in this chapter exercise was described as a means of opening communication between the mind and the physical self. Ayurvedic tradition teaches that this meeting between consciousness and physiology focuses itself at a number of vital locations on the body, known as *marma* points. Just as the flowing water of a river is deeper and swifter in certain areas, the energy produced by physical exertion gathers itself at these marmas. In all, there are 107 marma points, of which three are by far the most important. These three are places where the rivers of energy cross. Physical and psychic power flows through them to form the network of marma points throughout the body. These "great marmas" are known as *mahamarmas* in Sanskrit. One is located in the head, another in the lower abdominal region, and a third, called *hridaya-marma,* resides in the heart. Gentle exercises to stimulate hridayamarma can be of great benefit for healing the heart both physically and spiritually. The yoga poses described below are designed to have this effect.

Although many people in the West still associate yoga with difficult postures and ascetic lifestyles, this is a misunderstanding. Yoga, which means "union" in Sanskrit, is intended to bring the mind and the body together. Ideally, the poses are pathways to spiritual experience, not simply "exercises" in the athletic sense. Force, therefore, has no place in yoga, and any impulse toward straining to achieve a posture should be recognized as a step in the wrong direction. This is especially true for poses designed to benefit the heart. Practice these poses calmly and gently. There are many occasions throughout the day when hard work and competitiveness seem to be demanded. But yoga, properly understood, is about awareness rather than effort, and balance rather than diligent striving.

Toning-Up Exercise

This brief massage stimulates circulation and moves blood from the extremities toward the heart.

1. Sit comfortably with your back straight and your legs gently crossed. Using the palms and fingers of both hands, massage the top of your head, moving your hands slowly down toward your face, neck, and chest. Then start again at the top of your head, moving your hands down over the back of your neck and around to your chest.

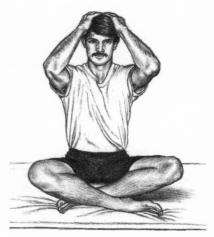

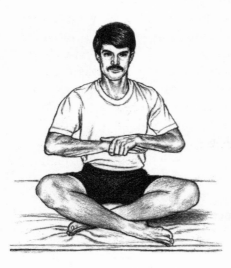

2. Now grasp the fingertips of your right hand with the palm and fingers of your left, gradually pressing and releasing your arm up to your shoulder and chest. Begin with the upper surface of your right arm, and then massage your left arm in the same way.

3. With the tips of your fingers meeting horizontally at your navel, begin to press and release your abdomen, gradually moving the pressure up toward the center of your chest.

4. Use both hands to press and release the middle of your back and ribs, moving up toward your heart as far as you can reach.

5. Starting with your right foot, massage the sole and the toes, gradually pressing and releasing up your calf, thigh, and waist. Repeat with your left foot.

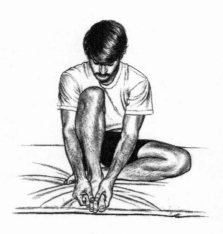

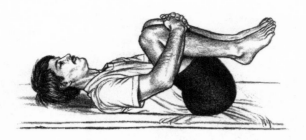

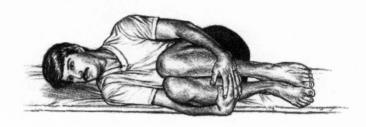

6. Lie on your back, draw your knees up to your chest, and clasp your hands over your knees. Raise your head slightly and roll to your right until your right wrist touches the floor. Then roll to the left. Repeat five times in each direction, then slowly extend your legs until you're lying on your back. Rest comfortably for at least a minute before sitting up.

Seated Twisting Pose (*Marichyasana*)

Marichyasana opens the chest area, deepens respiration, and stimulates the circulation of blood through the organs of the upper body, including the heart.

1. Begin by sitting comfortably with your legs outstretched. Now lift your left foot and place it flat on the floor.

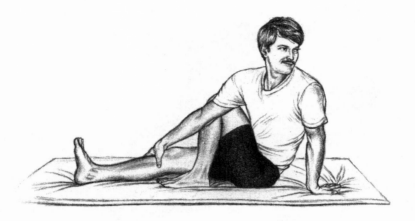

2. Place your left hand on the floor behind you, and press your right forearm against the outside of your left knee.
3. Inhale as deeply as comfort permits, then exhale as you twist from the base of your spine to the left, so that your chin moves back toward your left shoulder. Let the movement flow naturally from the exhalation of your breath.
4. Breathe normally as you hold this posture for a count of ten. With practice, you'll feel the depth of your breathing increase. Then slowly return to your starting position, with your legs outstretched. Now repeat the pose on the other side. Perform three cycles of the exercise in your beginning sessions, then gradually work up to seven.

Awareness Pose (*Chitasana*)

Despite the simplicity of this pose, *Chitasana* is extremely beneficial in developing mind/body awareness. As you perform this relaxing posture, let your attention move toward your chest area. Have the intention of healing your heart.

1. Begin by lying flat on your back. Allow your arms to
    rest easily by your side, with the palms up.
2. Close your eyes and let your whole body relax. As you
    breathe deeply and naturally, let your healing attention
    be drawn toward your heart.
3. Remain in this relaxed position for at least one minute,
    or longer if you choose. Then slowly open your eyes.

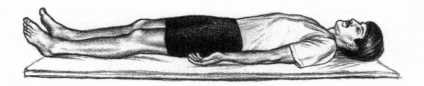

BUILDING CARDIOVASCULAR FITNESS

As you become comfortable with the breathing exercises and
yoga postures described in this chapter, you may choose to
gradually increase the intensity of your activity in order to
achieve a higher level of fitness.

This can have many benefits. After all, our bodies were
designed for movement. Over many thousands of years of
human history, people maintained a relatively high level of
physical activity. It's only in this century that large portions
of the population have had the option of "taking life easy."
Moreover, taking life *too* easy is often a mistake. Clinical
research since the 1950s has shown that active people have a
lower risk of coronary heart disease. And in people who have
already developed heart trouble, carefully controlled exercise
can improve quality of life, reduce the risk of more serious
illness, and even help reverse the damage that has already
been done.

Maintaining awareness of your body's internal signals is an essential element of building fitness. As you begin to get into shape, make it a habit to take your pulse before, during, and after any activity. For the first ninety days, it's best to gradually increase your exercise level so that your heart rate rises *not more* than 25 percent during the first month, and *up to* 50 percent for two months thereafter. For example, if your resting heart rate is 80 beats per minute, your pulse rate should stay below 96 for the first month, and should be no faster than 112 in the months that follow. Walking, light swimming, and bicycling are appropriate activities for this early stage of conditioning.

After three months of this relatively light aerobic exercise, you can step up the pace of your workouts to meet the recommended standards for your age group. Walking, swimming, and bicycling are still excellent conditioners, but you can now do them more briskly. Light jogging may also be appropriate.

It's best to aim for an average training heart rate that's 75 percent of your maximum. To find this number, first subtract your age from 220, then multiply the result by .75. For example, if you are 55 years old, your target heart rate during exercise can be calculated as follows:

$$220 - 55 = 165$$
$$165 \times .75 = 124 \; beats/minute$$

Most people find that an exercise program reaching this target rate provides optimal fitness benefits. The exercise should be performed three times a week, for 20 to 30 minutes per session. In addition, it's useful to keep the following points in mind:

• Each exercise session should include a light warm-up, an active period, and a cooling-down phase.
• During peak exercise, you may have a thin film of perspiration, but you should not be sweating profusely.

- You should easily be able to hold a conversation while exercising. If you're too short of breath to do so, reduce the intensity of your workout.
- Most important, emphasize activities that you enjoy.

The following precautions are recommended to maximize the benefits and minimize the risks associated with any cardiovascular fitness program:

- Wait at least 90 minutes after a meal before beginning exercise.
- Warm up and cool down slowly. Don't engage in sudden, vigorous activity.
- Don't exercise if you're not feeling well.
- **Stop and promptly notify your doctor if you experience chest discomfort, palpitations, or dizziness.**

Following is an outline for a 40-minute session combining meditation with physical exercise. This can serve as a model for your own program. Of course, you may choose to vary the length of the components to suit your own tastes, but the order of the activities should be retained:

1. Meditation: 10 minutes
2. Yoga postures with breathing awareness: 10 minutes
3. Aerobic activity: 20 minutes
4. Yoga postures: 5 minutes
5. Quiet resting: 5 minutes

9

MASSAGE

Perhaps you're not used to thinking of your skin as an organ of your body, but that's in fact what it is. The skin is the body's largest organ, and it is a rich source of healing substances. When stimulated by massage or another form of therapeutic touch, the skin produces antidepressants as well as powerful anti-cancer and anti-aging substances. Most important for our purposes here, the skin also produces hormones that facilitate healthy circulation and cardiac health.

Affection has enormous healing power, and in all living things touch is the sense that best expresses affection. The touch of a human hand on the body has immediate benefits for the emotions and, through them, for the physiology in general. Every neurochemical found in the nervous system is also present in the skin, and since touch can help stimulate the production of these substances, it's especially effective for calming the mind and for treating the anxiety and anger that have been implicated in coronary heart disease.

I'm quite fond of a certain study that demonstrates this principle. First published in 1970, over the years it's become known as something of a classic. Studying the causes of coronary heart disease, laboratory researchers fed an extremely high cholesterol diet to several groups of rabbits. But one technician who was feeding a group of these animals got into the habit of taking them out of their cages. He would pet the rabbits and cuddle them before feeding them their poisonous diet. Although this behavior was totally unauthorized, it turned out to be the most significant finding of the study. The rabbits that received affectionate treatment showed a significant decrease in atherosclerosis, and a much lower incidence of heart diseases of all kinds. The simple act of touching these animals totally transformed their bodies' ability to metabolize cholesterol.

This evidence has been supported by wide-ranging laboratory research on the many benefits of therapeutic touch. For example, massage releases growth hormones that help premature babies gain weight; it strengthens the immune system and elevates the emotions; it fosters the creation of natural pain relievers throughout the body and promotes relaxation and healthy sleep.

For thousands of years, Ayurveda has not only recognized the power of healing touch but has developed massage techniques for putting this power to use. Along with meditation, appropriate exercise, and a healthy diet, massage should be an important part of any program for preventing and reversing coronary heart disease.

MASSAGE AND THE DOSHAS

Massage can be gentle, or vigorous in order to reach deep tissues. Both the type of massage and the appropriate oil for you should be selected with an understanding of the needs of your physiology. Vata types, for example, with their tendencies toward worry and restlessness, benefit from a gentle massage using oils such as sesame or almond, which are heavy and warm.

Pitta types are prone to overheating and to heat-related conditions such as rashes and other skin problems. This same sensitivity to irritation is present in Pittas' coronary arteries. Pittas should use a deep massage with cooling oils such as coconut and olive.

Kapha types can become sedentary and sluggish when out of balance, so massage should serve as an energizing technique to counter these tendencies. Kaphas respond best to vigorous, stimulating massage using a light oil such as sunflower or safflower. Ayurvedic dry massage (see page 111) is also excellent for Kaphas.

ABHYANGA: OIL MASSAGE

An oil massage can be one of the most enjoyable parts of your daily routine. Known as *Abhyanga,* the full-body oil massage takes about ten minutes to perform. Abhyanga benefits the nervous and endocrine systems, enhances circulation, improves muscle tone, and stimulates the body's production of healing chemicals.

Preparing the Oil

- Cure massage oil once before you use it by slowly heating it in a glass or metal pot.
- Place a few drops of water in the oil. Then remove the pot from the heat as soon as the water boils out of the oil. Be sure to watch the oil carefully so that it doesn't begin to smoke and burn.
- Before performing the massage, the oil should be reheated above body temperature. To do this, put a small portion of oil in a plastic cup or squeeze bottle and place it in a bowl of hot water. Or microwave it for 10 to 15 seconds.

- The oil massage should be performed in the bathroom because some oil may spill. You may want to cover the floor with a large towel or plastic sheet.

Performing the Oil Massage

- Begin by pouring a tablespoon of warm oil on your scalp. Using circular motions, massage your head with the flat of your hand as if you were washing your hair, and then move to your face. Massage your forehead, and then move to your temples, again using circular motions. Then rub around the ears.
- Apply a little oil to your hands. Massage the front and back of your neck, using the flat of your hand and your fingers. Next, move to your shoulders.
- Massage your shoulders and then your arms, using circular motions at the joints and back-and-forth motions on the long parts.
- Now move to your chest and gently massage, using circular motions, then do the same to your stomach and lower abdomen.
- Without straining to reach, use up-and-down motions over your lower back and spine.
- Now vigorously massage the legs, moving back and forth on the long parts and using circular motions on the knees and ankles.
- Continue this vigorous massage onto your feet, using the flat of your hand except around the toes, which you can massage with your fingers.
- As you complete the massage there should be a thin, almost undetectable film of oil on your body. Gently wash yourself with warm (not hot) water and mild soap so you don't completely remove the oil.

Performing the Oil Mini-Massage

When there's not enough time for a full-body oil massage, you can perform an Ayurvedic mini-massage in just one or two minutes. This mini-massage focuses on the head and the feet, the parts of the body that will benefit most.

- To begin the oil mini-massage, pour a tablespoon of warm oil on your scalp. Massage your head with the flat of your hand, then move to your face. Massage your forehead and move to your temples, using circular motions. Then rub around the ears.
- With a second tablespoon of oil, massage the feet vigorously using the flat of your hand except around the toes, which you can massage with your fingers
- Now relax quietly for a few moments and soak in the oil. As with the full-body massage, wash gently with warm water and mild soap in order to leave a thin film of oil on your skin.

GARSHANA: DRY MASSAGE

Garshana, or dry massage, is best performed in the morning before bathing. It requires less than five minutes, and should be performed wearing special silk gloves, which are available from Ayurvedic sources (see page 147). Garshana stimulates circulation, and it is particularly good for stabilizing Kapha imbalances. Because Kapha is an inherently oily dosha, a dry massage such as Garshana is an excellent alternative to an oil massage. Garshana can also be used for pacifying unbalanced Pitta.

- To perform Garshana, begin by sitting on a stool or straight-backed chair. Then use both hands to massage your head in brisk circular motions.

- Shift to long strokes as you reach your neck and shoulders.
- Use circular motions at the shoulder joints, long strokes on your upper arms, then circular motions again at the elbows.
- Continue using long strokes down the lengths of your forearms, circular motions at the wrist, long strokes down the hands, and circular motions on the joints of your fingers.
- Now move to your chest. Massage horizontally with long strokes, though it's best to avoid direct massage over the heart and breasts.
- Massage your stomach using two horizontal strokes, followed by two diagonal strokes. Then alternate horizontal and diagonal strokes on the lower back, buttocks, and thighs. Give special attention to any area where extra fat is present, because massage can promote circulation and loosen toxins in these areas.
- Now stand up and use circular motions to massage your hip joints. Then massage your legs, using long strokes over the long bones and circular strokes at the knees and ankles. Complete your massage with long strokes over your feet.

NUTRITION FOR A

HEALTHY HEART

Our hearts—and all the other parts of our physical bodies—are created from the energy and information that we extract from the environment. This gathering of energy takes place in many ways; all our senses participate in it. But, along with breathing, taking in food is our most direct and intimate contact with the surrounding universe. The human digestive system, with its miraculous ability to assimilate nutrition and eliminate what is not needed, provides a dramatic display of biological intelligence.

In Ayurveda, sensible eating and strong digestion are the keys to good health. As we consume complex foods, they are broken down into the elemental nutritional components from which our cells and tissues are continuously being reconstructed. At every moment, we are literally transforming our own bodies through the exchange of raw material with the world around us. You are what you eat.

That a connection exists between diet and coronary heart

disease is beyond dispute. Yet the precise nature of that connection is by no means agreed upon, and new points of view keep emerging. At present, the general consensus is that individuals who consume large amounts of cholesterol and saturated (animal) fat are at greater risk for coronary heart disease.

Fats contribute to elevated levels of cholesterol in the blood, which may accumulate in blockages of the coronary arteries. Although less than 25 percent of the cholesterol in our bodies is derived from diet, what we eat does influence the volume of cholesterol in the bloodstream—and for the past hundred years or so, the influence has been largely in the wrong direction. Today, for example, Americans eat at least 50 percent more beef than at the beginning of the century. The American Heart Association recommends a diet in which no more than 30 percent of total calories are derived from fat, though some clinicians believe this is too lenient. In the typical American diet more than 40 percent of total calories are fat derived, exceeding even the AHA's relatively mild recommendations.

Current nutritional thinking strongly emphasizes reducing intake of fat. In its place, consumption of vegetables, fruits, and bran is encouraged, since diets emphasizing these elements have been shown to reduce blood cholesterol levels by as much as 20 percent. There is also evidence that antioxidants found in fresh fruits and vegetables may slow the development of coronary artery disease.

MINDFULNESS IN EATING

Eating with mindfulness means, first, selecting food that meets your individual needs, both physically and emotionally. The food should be prepared in a nourishing way, and it should be eaten in a setting that promotes optimal digestion. By following the Body Intelligence Techniques listed below, you can enhance your enjoyment of a meal so that it's both heart healthy and delicious.

Body Intelligence Techniques

- **Eat only when you are hungry, and don't eat until your last meal has been digested.** This usually takes from three to six hours.
- **Whenever possible, eat freshly cooked meals.** Both raw foods and leftovers are often difficult to digest. Certain uncooked foods, such as salads, are fine, but in general Ayurveda recommends well-cooked meals.
- **Eat in a quiet, relaxed atmosphere.** Even if you have only 15 or 20 minutes for your meal, it's important to set everything else aside and allow your body to focus on eating and digesting. This can't happen amid noise and distractions.
- **Always eat sitting down and at a moderate pace.** This helps focus awareness and increases enjoyment of food.
- **Don't eat when you're upset.** If you're angry or nervous, put off eating until you feel calmer.
- **Avoid overeating.** Ayurveda teaches that we should eat to only three-quarters of our capacity. More than this smothers the digestive fire.
- **Avoid cold foods and iced drinks.** These chill the system and create toxic accumulations. In fact, sipping warm water while you eat can soothe the gastrointestinal tract and facilitate digestion.
- **Chew food thoroughly.** This makes digestion easier, and enhances your awareness of how each food tastes.
- **Take a few minutes to rest after you eat.** This helps digestion begin without stress.

THE SIX TASTES

Every bite of food delivers vast amounts of information to your system. The human body can perceive a sweet taste in a dilution of 1 part to 200—and a bitter taste in a dilution of 1 part to 2 million!

Ayurveda recognizes six tastes. *Sweet, sour, salty,* and *bitter* are readily familiar, but *pungent* and *astringent* may be less so. Pungent foods, such as salsa, are hot and spicy, while astringent foods, such as pomegranates and beans, cause a puckering sensation in your mouth.

Ideally, all six tastes should be included in every meal. But your mind/body type, as well as the current condition of your health, may make it beneficial to emphasize one taste over another. Keep this in mind as you read over the dietary recommendations for stabilizing the three doshas, which are presented below. These are intended to balance healthy nutritional principles with your individual needs.

EATING FOR HEALTH AND BALANCE

Ayurveda recommends following a diet that meets the needs of your dominant dosha when your system is in balance, or that pacifies an unbalanced dosha. The dietary suggestions in this section are for these purposes.

Although Vata imbalance is highly stressful and can be dangerous for the heart and to overall health, most coronary heart disease arises out of Pitta or Kapha imbalances. Please pay particular attention to the suggestions for stabilizing those two doshas.

Vata-Balancing Diet

Vata is dry, cold, light, and above all unpredictable. To stabilize Vata, emphasize foods that are warm and substantial.

GENERAL RECOMMENDATIONS:
- Emphasize foods that are warm, heavy, oily and thoroughly cooked. Minimize foods that are cold, dry, light, and raw.
- Emphasize sweet, sour, and salty tastes. Minimize pungent, bitter, and astringent.
- Eat larger quantities, but not more than you can digest easily.

SPECIFIC RECOMMENDATIONS:
- Dairy: All dairy products pacify Vata.
- Sweeteners: All sweeteners are good (in moderation) for pacifying Vata.
- Oils: All oils pacify Vata.
- Grains: Rice and wheat are excellent. Reduce barley, corn, millet, buckwheat, rye, and oats.
- Fruits: Emphasize sweet, sour, or heavy fruits, such as oranges, bananas, avocados, grapes, cherries, peaches, melons, berries, plums, pineapples, mangoes, and papayas. Reduce dry or light fruits, such as apples, pears, pomegranates, cranberries, and dried fruits.
- Vegetables: Beets, cucumbers, carrots, asparagus, and sweet potatoes are good. They should be cooked, not raw. The following vegetables are acceptable in moderate quantities if they're cooked, especially with ghee or Vata-reducing spices: peas, broccoli, cauliflower, celery, zucchini, and green leafy vegetables. It's better to avoid sprouts and cabbage.
- Nuts: All nuts are good.
- Beans: Reduce all beans, except tofu and split–mung bean soup.
- Spices: Cardamom, cumin, ginger, cinnamon, salt, cloves, mustard seed, and small quantities of black pepper are good.
- Meat and fish (for nonvegetarians): Chicken, turkey, and seafood are acceptable; beef should be avoided.

Pitta-Balancing Diet

Because coronary heart disease is fundamentally an inflammatory condition, Pitta's association with heat makes stabilizing this dosha particularly important. A Pitta-balancing diet should cool the system, while avoiding foods that are hot or spicy.

GENERAL RECOMMENDATIONS:
- Emphasize foods that are cool or warm. Minimize foods that are steaming hot in temperature.
- Emphasize sweet, bitter, and astringent tastes. Minimize pungent, salty, and sour.

SPECIFIC RECOMMENDATIONS:
- Dairy: Milk, butter, and ghee are good for pacifying Pitta. Reduce yogurt, cheese, sour cream, and cultured buttermilk (as their sour tastes aggravate Pitta). Egg yolk increases Pitta and should be avoided.
- Sweeteners: All sweeteners are good except honey and molasses.
- Oils: Olive, sunflower, and coconut oils are best. Reduce sesame, almond, and corn oil, all of which increase Pitta.
- Grains: Wheat, white rice, barley, and oats are good. Reduce corn, rye, millet, and brown rice.
- Fruits: Emphasize sweet fruits, such as grapes, cherries, melons, berries, avocados, coconuts, pomegranates, mangoes, and sweet, fully ripened oranges, pineapples, and plums. Reduce sour fruits, such as grapefruits, olives, papayas, persimmons, and sour unripe oranges, pineapples, and plums.
- Vegetables: Emphasize asparagus, cucumbers, potatoes, sweet potatoes, pumpkins, broccoli, cauliflower, celery,

okra, lettuce, green beans, zucchini, and green leafy vegetables, such as lettuce. Reduce hot peppers, tomatoes,
carrots, beets, onions, garlic, radishes, spinach, and mustard greens.

- Beans: Reduce all beans, except tofu and split–mung
bean soup.
- Spices: Cinnamon, coriander, cardamom, and fennel are
good. But the following spices strongly increase Pitta and
should be eaten only in small amounts: ginger, cumin,
black pepper, fenugreek, cloves, celery seed, salt, and mustard seed. Chili peppers and cayenne should be avoided.
- Meat and fish (for nonvegetarians): Chicken, pheasant,
and turkey are preferable. Beef and seafood increase Pitta
and should be avoided.

Kapha-Balancing Diet

Kapha is a cold and moist dosha, related to the elements of earth
and water. Kapha-balancing foods are light, warm, and spicy,
to counter Kapha's tendency toward heaviness and inertia.

GENERAL RECOMMENDATIONS:
- Emphasize foods that are light, dry, and warm. Minimize
foods that are heavy, oily, and cold.
- Keep breakfasts and dinners light, emphasizing lightly
cooked foods, raw fruits, and vegetables.
- Emphasize pungent, bitter, and astringent tastes. Minimize sweet, salty, and sour.

SPECIFIC RECOMMENDATIONS:
- Dairy: In general, avoid dairy products, except low-fat
milk.
- Sweeteners: Honey is excellent for reducing Kapha. Reduce
sugar products, as these increase Kapha.

- Grains: Most grains are fine, especially barley and millet. Avoid wheat and rice, as they increase Kapha.
- Fruit: Lighter fruits, such as apples and pears, are best. Reduce heavy or sour fruits, such as oranges, bananas, pineapples, figs, dates, avocados, coconuts, and melons, as these fruits increase Kapha.
- Vegetables: All are fine, except tomatoes, cucumbers, sweet potatoes, and zucchini, as they increase Kapha.
- Beans: All beans are fine except soybeans (including tofu and tempeh products), which increase Kapha.
- Oils: Since all oils increase Kapha, which is a naturally oily dosha, their use should be minimized.
- Nuts: Reduce all nuts.
- Spices: All spices are good except salt, which should be avoided, as it increases Kapha.
- Meat and fish (for nonvegetarians): White meat from chicken or turkey is fine, as is seafood. Reduce red meat.

	TO BALANCE VATA	TO BALANCE PITTA	TO BALANCE KAPHA
GENERAL	Favor warm, heavier	Favor cooler	Favor lighter
SIX TASTES	More sweet, sour, salty Less pungent, bitter, astringent	More sweet, bitter, astringent Less pungent, sour, salty	More pungent, bitter, astringent Less sweet, sour, salty
GRAINS	Rice, wheat	White rice, wheat, barley, oats	Most grains, especially barley and millet
DAIRY	Favor all	Reduce yogurt	Reduce all, except low-fat milk
OILS	Favor all	Olive, sunflower, coconut	Reduce all
BEANS	Mung beans, tofu	Reduce all	All beans, except soy beans

	TO BALANCE VATA	TO BALANCE PITTA	TO BALANCE KAPHA
VEGETABLES	Reduce sprouts, cabbage	Reduce tomatoes, onions, radishes	Reduce tomatoes, cucumbers, sweet potatoes, zucchini
FRUITS	Sweet, sour, heavy	Reduce sour	Reduce sour, heavy
SPICES	Ginger, cumin, cinnamon, cardamom, salt, cloves, mustard seed, black pepper	Reduce ginger, cumin, fenugreek, celery seed, black pepper, cloves, mustard seed, salt	Reduce salt

WEIGHT CONTROL

If you are overweight, there is much evidence that your risk of coronary heart disease is increased. But as in all aspects of Ayurveda, the process of arriving at a healthy weight involves learning to listen to your own needs. Just as you shouldn't let your ideal weight be dictated by an arbitrary chart or a culturally imposed standard of attractiveness, the process by which you attain your goals should also be a personal decision.

When I decided to lose twenty-five pounds, I was greatly helped by the program presented in *The Zone,* the best-selling book by Barry Sears, Ph.D. Minimizing carbohydrates while emphasizing fruits and vegetables wasn't difficult for me, and I appreciated the fact that fats did not have to be radically reduced. As an endocrinologist, I was also interested in Dr. Sears's comments on a little-known class of hormones called *eicosanoids,* which may have powerful disease-fighting properties. You might also respond well to the ideas put forward in *The Zone,* or you might find that an entirely different approach works better for you.

No matter what technique you use to control your weight, however, an Ayurvedic principle I mentioned earlier in this chapter is universally beneficial. This is *mindfulness*. In this context, mindfulness means you should eat whenever you experience a genuine sensation of hunger, but you should not eat when you really want something other than food, such as companionship, an outlet for anger, or relief from boredom.

Keeping a written record of your eating-related behaviors is an excellent way of bringing mindfulness into the eating area of your life. Draw up a simple chart indicating the hours of the day, and then estimate your hunger levels at 60-minute intervals. Use a scale of 1 to 10. At the bottom of the page, write down what you ate at each meal during the day and the times the meals were eaten. Include any snacks.

Each morning, glance at your chart for the previous few days. If you see any patterns you want to change, do so. Even if you don't make any conscious changes, merely keeping these written records will begin to positively affect your eating habits. Here, as always, self-awareness is the first and most important step toward health.

11

HEART-HEALTHY RECIPES

The recipes provided below are by no means intended as a comprehensive listing of the almost infinite variety of healthy dishes that can be prepared easily and affordably. But whether you're just beginning to cook "for your heart," or you're already a heart-wise chef, these recipes are sure to please.

I'm very grateful to Ginna Bell Bragg, co-author of *A Simple Celebration: A Vegetarian Cookbook for Body, Mind, and Spirit,* for her help with this chapter. Please note that Bragg's Liquid Aminos, an unfermented soy sauce used in several of the following recipes, is a commercial product that has no association with Ginna Bell Bragg.

GHEE

Ghee is an essential ingredient in Ayurvedic cooking. It is easy to digest and contributes to the absorption of nutrients. It can be purchased in most health food and Indian food stores. But buying it is expensive. Once you make your own, and discover how simple and delicious it is, you'll never buy it again.

1 or more pounds sweet, unsalted butter *(organic, if possible)*

1. Cut butter into cubes and cook at medium high heat in a heavy saucepan until melted. The butter will begin to foam and become white and frothy, making cracking and popping sounds. This is caused by the evaporation of moisture. Allow to bubble in this way for about ten minutes, or until cracking noises subside.

2. The next part of the process must be done carefully. As the cooking continues, the butter will foam up a second time as the milk solids begin to separate and turn golden brown. When the solids are browned, turn off the heat and let stand for about fifteen minutes to allow the ghee to cool. Pour into jars, straining the ghee through cheesecloth. Throw the solids away.

3. Store in airtight containers for up to three months in a refrigerator or six weeks at room temperature.

GRANOLA

Because this granola is made without butter or added sugar, it is healthful and nutritious.

    2 cups organic rolled oats
    ¼ cup sesame seeds
    ¼ cup sunflower seeds
    ¼ cup nuts, such as chopped almonds, chopped walnuts,
        or pine nuts
    2 tablespoons cinnamon
    1 teaspoon cardamom
    2 tablespoons grated orange peel

½ cup apple or orange juice concentrate
½ cup date pieces
½ cup raisins or currants
½ cup dried mixed fruit pieces
½ cup coconut, optional

Preheat oven to 325. Combine the oats, seeds, nuts, spices, and orange peel in mixing bowl. Mix well. Add juice concentrate and mix. Spread mixture on baking sheets. Bake for about 45 minutes, stirring frequently, until toasted and dry. Allow to cool before adding fruits and coconut. Omit coconut and nuts for a lower-fat granola. Store in an airtight container.

PLAIN MUESLI

If served with nonfat milk or yogurt, this is a great fat-free breakfast.

2 cups organic rolled oats

Preheat oven to 325. Spread oats on baking sheet. Bake for about 45 minutes, stirring frequently, until toasted and dry. Allow to cool. Store in an airtight container.

BAKED APPLE

Simple and delicious, a baked apple is great for breakfast or dessert. This recipe can also be used with pears.

1 pippin or Granny Smith apple
½ teaspoon ghee
2 teaspoons ground pine nuts
1 teaspoon maple syrup
¼ cup apple juice

(continued on next page)

Peel top of apple, about ⅓ of the way down. Cut out center core, leaving a well about 1 inch in diameter. Mix ghee, pine nuts, and maple syrup and fill well of apple. Place in baking dish with apple juice. Cover with foil and bake about 30 minutes. Uncover, baste with apple juice, and bake until soft, about 15 minutes.

WHOLE-WHEAT CHAPATI

A good, yeast-free bread.

> 2¼ cups whole-wheat pastry flour
> 2 teaspoons sunflower or canola oil
> 1¼ cups lukewarm water with pinch of salt
> Extra flour for rolling

1. With a wooden spoon, mix flour and oil in a large bowl. Add water and mix into a soft dough. Cover and let stand for an hour.
2. Moisten your hands with oil and make 25–30 small balls. Roll balls in small bowl of flour. Using rolling pin, roll out on a floured surface to form 6-inch circles.
3. Heat large skillet or griddle to medium. Cook chapatis 30 seconds on first side, about 1 minute on second side, until they puff. Serve immediately or keep covered until ready to use.

FRENCH BREAD

This is a favorite at the Chopra Center. Try different flour and flavoring combinations. The variations are endless.

> 2 tablespoons yeast
> 2 tablespoons raw sugar
> 4 cups lukewarm water

8 cups sifted organic, unbleached white flour or mixture of
white and whole-wheat pastry flour

½ tablespoon sea salt

1. Dissolve yeast and sugar in 2 cups water. Let stand for ten
   minutes. Stir into flour and salt. Add just enough of the rest
   of the water to hold dough together—it will form a soft,
   sticky dough. Knead in bowl for about 5 minutes. Cover
   and let rise for 2–4 hours. (If you set dough near a warm
   stove or oven, it will rise faster.) When risen, punch down
   and divide into loaves—two medium loaf pans, or one
   large one. Clay pans are best. Let rise again for 25 minutes,
   or until risen over the top of the pan.
2. Bake at 400 for about 40 minutes, or until browned and
   crusty. Add Italian herbs to dry flour for a Tuscan flavor.

BRUSCHETTA

*This is best during late summer/early fall, in tomato season.
Buy organic, fresh tomatoes and taste the difference.*

1 pound fresh, vine-ripened Roma tomatoes, chopped and
   drained

1 garlic clove, minced

1 tablespoon scallions, minced

Juice of one lemon

1 teaspoon lemon zest

1 cup fresh basil, minced

8 slices bread or one focaccia

¼ cup olive oil, optional

Blend first six ingredients in small bowl. Refrigerate until an
hour before serving. Toast bread or focaccia, brushing with
olive oil before toasting or baking (optional) Serve warm toast
or focaccia with bowls of bruschetta for topping.

HUMMUS DIP

This version of Middle Eastern hummus has no oil added. Oil adds many calories.

> 3 cups cooked chickpeas
> ¼ to ½ cup orange juice (concentrate may be used for
>   more intense flavor)
> ¼ cup sesame seeds
> Juice of one lemon
> 1 teaspoon Bragg's Liquid Aminos
> 1 clove garlic (optional)
> Paprika, to taste
> 1 teaspoon fresh cilantro

Place chickpeas in food processor and process for 3 minutes at high speed. Orange juice may be added if paste becomes too thick to process. Add remaining ingredients and process until smooth. Refrigerate until one hour before serving. Serve with pita bread or lavosh.

MUSHROOM SPINACH SOUP WITH SHERRY

As with all soups, fresh homemade stock adds deep flavor.

> 2 yellow onions, chopped
> 1 tablespoon olive oil
> 1 clove garlic, chopped
> 1 pound mushrooms, chopped
> 1 bunch spinach, chopped
> 2 carrots, grated
> 2 tablespoons tarragon
> 1 teaspoon salt

3 tablespoons Bragg's Liquid Aminos
6 cups rich vegetable stock*
¼ cup sherry

Sauté onions and garlic in olive oil over medium heat until soft. Add mushrooms and simmer one minute. Add spinach, carrots, tarragon, salt, Bragg's Liquid Aminos, and stock. Bring to boil. Remove from heat. Add sherry. Reheat before serving.

CURRIED TEMPEH SALAD

This salad tastes so much like chicken, it will fool the most resolute meat-eater.

2 packages tempeh, steamed and crumbled
3 tablespoons cilantro, minced
3 tablespoons fresh parsley, chopped
¼ cup almonds, chopped
¼ cup raisins or currants
¼ cup celery, chopped
1 teaspoon turmeric
1 teaspoon garam masala, consisting of coriander, cumin, cardamom, and cinnamon
1 tablespoon Bragg's Liquid Aminos
¼ cup nonfat yogurt
⅛ teaspoon salt

Combine all ingredients in large bowl. Toss well. Roll into lavosh (flat, unleavened bread) or shape into rounds on a bed of lettuce. Garnish with parsley.

---

*Stock can be made at home by bringing six cups water to boil with three pounds of vegetable scrapings or fresh vegetables. Simmer for 2–6 hours.

KALAMATA PASTA SALAD

This is a quickie for after work or unexpected guests. Keep ingredients on hand in your pantry.

2 pounds fresh pasta, any shape, cooked
1 teaspoon olive oil
1 tablespoon dry onion flakes
1 clove garlic, chopped
¼ cup pepitas*
½ cup golden raisins, chopped
¼ cup Kalamata olives, pitted
¼ cup celery, chopped
¼ cup fresh basil, chopped
½ cup grated carrots

Dressing:

⅛ cup oil from sun-dried tomatoes
1 tablespoon Bragg's Liquid Aminos
Dash balsamic vinegar
1 teaspoon honey
1 teaspoon lemon juice
Salt and pepper to taste

Sauté onions, garlic, pepitas, celery, raisins, and olives in olive oil for 2 minutes. Toss with remaining ingredients. Combine ingredients for dressing and add to pasta. Serve at room temperature.

*This pumpkin-like seed comes from Mexico, and is available in health food stores.

LENTIL-RICE SALAD

Lentils and rice together create a complete protein. Serve this dish on a warm day with tomato chutney and chapati (unleavened bread, much like a tortilla).

3 cups cooked brown or green lentils, cooled
1 cup cooked basmati rice, cooled
1 cup chopped celery
1 cup carrots
1 cup cooked peas, cooled (if using frozen peas, choose organic, if possible, and do not cook)
2 tablespoons scallions, finely chopped
¼ cup parsley, chopped

Mustard Dressing:

2 tablespoons Dijon mustard
1 tablespoon olive oil
1 tablespoon honey
1 tablespoon Bragg's Liquid Aminos
1 tablespoon lemon juice
½ cup orange juice

Blanch carrots by immersing in boiling water for 5 minutes. Remove from pot and immediately rinse with cold water to stop cooking and retain color; when cool, chop. Combine all ingredients except dressing in bowl and gently toss with mustard dressing.

VEGETABLE TART

Vary the vegetables to make this tart unique each time you create it.

1 large leek, washed, chopped, and washed again
1 cup grated carrots
1 pound spinach
1 cup toasted pine nuts, ground
1 pound firm tofu
2 tablespoons Bragg's Liquid Aminos
1 teaspoon tarragon
4 eggs
½ cup bread crumbs
2 tablespoons sesame seeds

1. Preheat oven to 400°.
2. In dry, nonstick pan, sauté leeks, carrots, and spinach for 2 minutes.
3. Blend vegetables with pine nuts and tofu in food processor until finely ground or chopped.
4. Combine mixture with remaining ingredients (except sesame seeds) in a large bowl. Pour into an oiled or sprayed 9x12-inch baking dish and sprinkle with sesame seeds.
5. Bake, uncovered, for 30 minutes. Serves 6 to 8.

BAKED WINTER SQUASH WITH
WILD RICE–CRANBERRY STUFFING

This is a luscious holiday main course or side dish. It's filled with goodies.

2 medium winter squash (kabocha, acorn, golden nugget, butternut)
1 cup orange juice
1 cup wild rice
2 cups water
Pinch salt
½ cup toasted pine nuts
¼ cup dried cranberries
1 tablespoon dried onion flakes
1 teaspoon grated orange peel
1 tablespoon Bragg's Liquid Aminos
1 teaspoon dried sage
2 tablespoons bread crumbs

1. Preheat oven to 350°. Split squash in half lengthwise. Remove seeds and stringy pulp with large spoon. Place in baking dish with orange juice; cover and bake for 45 minutes, until cooked but still firm. Reserve juice.
2. Bring 2 cups water to boil. Add rice and salt. Simmer for 30–40 minutes, until rice is fluffy.
3. Combine rice with remaining ingredients, except bread crumbs. Insert filling in the hollow of the squash. Add reserved orange juice to filling.
4. Sprinkle with bread crumbs. Bake for 30 minutes, until heated through and bread crumbs are browned.

CHEESELESS LASAGNA

For a dairy-free diet, this is a winner. The sun-dried tomatoes give intense flavor.

One package spinach lasagna noodles, cooked and drained
Bread crumbs

Sauce:

6 carrots, peeled and sliced
6 zucchini, sliced
6 stalks celery, chopped
1 teaspoon ghee
One bunch parsley
1 16-oz. jar sun-dried tomatoes, drained
1 tablespoon oregano
Dash salt
⅛ teaspoon Italian seasoning

Filling:

1 package hard-style tofu, crumbled
1½ cups sauce
½ cup pine nuts, ground

1. Sauté carrots, zucchini, and celery in ghee for 5 minutes. Combine with rest of sauce ingredients and grind coarsely in food processor. Return to pot and simmer for 5 minutes.
2. Combine filling ingredients.
3. Layer in casserole dish in the following order: sauce, noodles, filling; sauce, noodles, filling; sauce, noodles, sauce, bread crumbs.
4. Bake at 350° uncovered for 40 minutes, or until bread crumbs are golden and lasagna is bubbling.

MINTED PEA SOUFFLÉ

This works as a main or side dish. Try a dollop of nonfat yogurt blended with mint for a topping.

2 medium shallots, chopped
½ teaspoon ghee
1 pound fresh peas
2 eggs, beaten
½ cup ricotta cheese
Pinch tarragon
1 teaspoon fresh or dried mint
Pinch of salt
2 tablespoons Bragg's Liquid Aminos
¼ cup fresh bread crumbs

1. In a skillet, sauté shallots in ghee until tender. Add peas and continue to cook for three minutes.
2. In food processor, puree peas and shallots. Mix well with eggs, ricotta, tarragon, mint, salt, and Bragg's Liquid Aminos.
3. Pour into oiled casserole dish. Sprinkle with bread crumbs.
4. Bake at 350° until firm and bread crumbs are browned, about 30 minutes. Serves 4 to 6.

RED LENTIL DHAL

*This dhal is rich and full of aromatic aromas. It will entice
your family into the kitchen to see "what's cooking."*

>1 quart dry red lentils
>Vegetable stock to cover lentils, plus 4 inches
>⅛ cup cumin, ground
>2 tablespoons turmeric
>2 tablespoons ghee
>2 tablespoons mustard seeds
>2 tablespoons cumin seeds
>Generous pinch whole fenugreek
>5 whole cardamom pods
>3 cinnamon sticks
>Generous pinch asafetida*
>1 cup leeks, chopped
>⅛ cup coriander
>2 tablespoons ground cardamom
>2-inch piece fresh ginger, finely chopped
>1 cup golden raisins, chopped
>Chopped cilantro for garnish
>2 tablespoons tomato paste
>½ tablespoon salt

1. Bring lentils to boil in pressure cooker, uncovered. Skim
   foam from top until foam subsides. Add ground cumin and
   turmeric. Simmer.
2. Heat ghee in skillet. Add mustard seeds, cumin seeds, fenugreek, cardamom pods, and cinnamon sticks. Let seeds siz-
   zle and pop. Add asafetida and leeks. Sauté until soft.
3. Add remaining spices and raisins. Sauté 5 minutes. Add ½
   cup water and tomato paste. Continue cooking 5 minutes.

---

*This Ayurvedic spice, which resembles garlic and contributes to digestion,
can be found in health food and Indian stores.

4. Add spice mixture to lentils. Cover with pressure cooker lid. When pressure top pops, reduce heat to low. Cook for 1 hour.

5. Turn off heat. When pressure top falls back down, open and taste. More coriander may be added at end. Garnish with cilantro.

CAROB TAHINI NUGGETS

Energy boosters! Pack them in your lunch or take on a trip.

½ cup pine nuts
¼ cup sunflower seeds
½ cup raisins or dried cranberries
½ cup sesame tahini butter
¼ cup unsweetened coconut
2 tablespoons carob powder
3 tablespoons maple syrup
Extra unsweetened coconut for rolling

Place nuts, seeds, and dried fruit in food processor and process for one minute, until chopped well. Add tahini, coconut, and carob powder. Process for 1 minute, dripping maple syrup through top hole. This will create a sticky "dough." Roll dough to form 1-inch balls. Roll in extra coconut. Form squares or rectangles or balls. Refrigerate in airtight container to set. Keep refrigerated.

BLUEBERRY BLISS BALLS

These are a favorite energy source for between meals or as a light dessert. They are not low-fat, so enjoy but don't overdo!

1 cup dried blueberries
½ cup pine nuts
½ cup unsweetened coconut
¼ cup sunflower seeds
2 teaspoons maple syrup
¼ cup unsweetened coconut for rolling

Place the first four ingredients in food processor and process for thirty seconds at high speed or until finely chopped. Pour in maple syrup and process for additional 20 seconds. Scoop out one teaspoon at a time, form into balls, and roll in coconut. Refrigerate for at least a half hour to firm balls. Store in an airtight container in the refrigerator.

ZIPPY ALMONDS

Almonds are sweet and slightly bitter. Soak them overnight to increase digestibility. These almonds have a spicy, fiery flavor—great to boost the appetite.

2 cups whole almonds, soaked overnight and dried
½ teaspoon ghee or olive oil
1 clove garlic, minced or crushed
1 teaspoon Bragg's Liquid Aminos
1 teaspoon chili flakes, or ½ teaspoon chili paste
1 teaspoon turbinado sugar

Sauté almonds in medium-hot ghee or oil for five minutes, stirring frequently. Add garlic, Bragg's Liquid Aminos, chili flakes or paste, and sugar. Toss to coat almonds. Turn off heat and let stand for ten minutes, until completely cooled. May be stored in an airtight container for several weeks.

12

THE CHOICE OF A

HEALING HEART

Prakriti is one of the most impor-
tant words in the Ayurvedic tradition. It refers to your true,
unique nature, the *self* that you were at the moment of your
birth. Nature intends for each of us to live in accordance with
our prakriti, not because it represents any rigidly ordained
destiny, but because prakriti is the fulfillment of the unique
strengths and vulnerabilities that express themselves in every
person who is now alive, or who has ever lived.

Another Sanskrit word, *vikriti,* denotes the deviations from
our true nature that occur during the course of our lives. Illness is a physical expression of vikriti, just as unhappiness is
its emotional manifestation. My purpose in this book has been
to show the inextricably close relationship between those two
negative qualities, and to suggest ways they can be replaced by
wellness and joy.

Vikriti is inevitable in this world, but your prakriti is within
your reach as well. You can always regain the wondrous power
that was yours as a child. You can always relearn what you

came into the world already knowing how to do. Starting today, you can once again begin to see the world as new. And by opening your eyes in this way, you can heal your heart.

Direct experience of the natural world is one of the best ways to recapture the wonder of life. For example:

- Walk barefoot for at least ten minutes every day. Have the intention to absorb the energy of the earth.
- Walk beside a natural body of water. Allow the cooling, cohering quality of water to infuse your being.
- Feel the light and warmth of the sun. Acknowledge the energy-giving power of the source of all life.
- Take a walk in an area of abundant vegetation, and deeply inhale the healing breath of plants. The ideal time to receive the life force of plants is shortly before dawn, and just after sunset.
- At night, gaze up at the stars. Let your awareness extend to the limits of the universe.

Can such simple activities as these really be the path to health? Yes—but there are many paths to health. If you are confronting coronary heart disease, I am not suggesting that you forsake modern medical treatment in favor of spiritual exploration. They work best together. Indeed, in the preceding chapters I've tried to present a balanced appraisal of contemporary treatments in order to help you take best advantage of them. But there are many books on coronary heart disease that can do that for you. What sets the Ayurvedic approach apart—and what can set you apart in dealing with CHD—is the realization that healing power is not found in any machine or medication. With the elegance and intelligence that characterizes all her works, Nature has placed the strength to heal this dreaded illness in the very same location as the disease itself. Both that strength and that vulnerability are, quite literally, *in our hearts*. We have only to choose between them.

But I know you've already made your choice. And my heart goes out to yours.

BIBLIOGRAPHY

Bragg, Ginna Bell, and David Simon, M.D. *A Simple Celebration*. New York: Harmony Books, 1996.

Carlson, Karen J., Stephanie A. Eisenstat, and Terra Ziporyn. *The Harvard Guide to Women's Health*. Cambridge, Mass.: Harvard University Press, 1996.

Chopra, Deepak. *Ageless Body, Timeless Mind*. New York: Harmony Books, 1993.

Harrison's Principles of Internal Medicine, 13th ed. New York: McGraw-Hill, 1994.

Lonsdorf, Nancy, M.D., Veronica Butler, M.D., and Melanie Brown. *A Woman's Best Medicine*. New York: Jeremy P. Tarcher/Putnam, 1993.

Love, Susan M., M.D., with Karen Lindsey. *Dr. Susan Love's Hormone Book*. New York: Random House, 1997.

McGoon, Michael D., M.D. *The Mayo Clinic Heart Book.* New York: William Morrow, 1993.

Ornish, Dean, M.D. *Dr. Dean Ornish's Program for Reversing Heart Disease.* New York: Ballantine Books, 1990.

Simon, David, M.D. *The Wisdom of Healing.* New York: Harmony Books, 1997.

Stohecker, James, ed. *Alternative Medicine.* Puyallup, Wash.: Future Medicine Publishing, 1994.

Whitaker, Julian M., M.D. *Reversing Heart Disease.* New York: Warner Books, 1985.

ACKNOWLEDGMENTS

For additional information on Ayurveda, mind/body medicine, and programs and treatments offered by The Chopra Center for Well Being, please contact:

The Chopra Center for Well Being
7630 Fay Avenue
La Jolla, CA 92037
(888) 424-6772 (toll free)
(619) 551-7788

I am very grateful to my colleague, David Simon, M.D., for his work on the questionnaires in chapters 3 and 4.

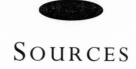

SOURCES

More information on Mind/Body and Ayurvedic treatments, products, herbs, and educational programs can be obtained from the following organizations:

The Chopra Center for Well Being
7630 Fay Avenue
La Jolla, CA 92037
(800) 257-8897 or (619) 551-7788
Fax: (619) 551-7825

Ayurvedic Institute
1311 Menaul N.E., Suite A 11311
Albuquerque, NM 87112
(505) 291-9698
Fax: (505) 294-7572

American Institute of Vedic Studies
P.O. Box 8357
Santa Fe, NM 87504

American School of Ayurvedic Science
10025 N.E. 4th Street
Bellevue, WA 98004

Maharishi Ayurved Products
Colorado Springs, CO
(800) 255-8332

INDEX

ABOUT THE AUTHOR

Deepak Chopra, M.D., is a distinguished writer, lecturer, and physician. He has written nineteen books, which have been translated into thirty-five languages. He is also the author of more than thirty audio and videotape series, including five critically acclaimed works on public television: *Body, Mind, and Soul; The Seven Spiritual Laws of Success; The Way of the Wizard; The Crystal Cave;* and *Alchemy*. Dr. Chopra currently serves as director for education programs at The Chopra Center for Well Being in La Jolla, California.

Deepak Chopra and The Chopra Center for Well Being in La Jolla, California, offer a wide range of seminars, products, and educational programs worldwide. The Chopra Center offers revitalizing mind/body programs, as well as day spa services. Guests can come to rejuvenate, expand knowledge, or obtain a medical consultation.

For information on meditation classes, health and well-being courses, instructor certification programs, or local classes in